Contents

List of Illustrations | viii

Acknowledgements | ix

Part I Society Dances
1 Fashionable Bodies and Society Dancing | 3
2 Fashioning Dance Histories | 13
3 The Seasonal Round | 22
4 Public Spaces | 35
5 Late Victorian Repertoire | 46
6 Anarchy in the Ball Room | 58

Part II Fashioning Gentility
7 A Noble Profession | 75
8 Temples of Terpsichore | 86
9 The Fashioning of Ladies | 95
10 Modelling the Lady | 111
11 Where Are Our Men? | 118
12 Dancing Dogs and Manly Men | 128

Part III Modern Moves
13 Moving into the Twentieth Century | 141
14 Modernizing Terpsichore | 149
15 Civilization Under Threat | 160
16 Knuts and Aliens | 170
17 Civilizing from the Centre | 182
18 Looking Back, Moving On | 195

Appendix: Key Personnel in Society Dancing in England 1870–1920 | 201

Notes | 207

Bibliography | 224

Index | 238

List of Illustrations

3.1 A State Ball at Buckingham Palace, 1870   25

3.2 Dance Card, Late Nineteenth Century   31

4.1 Excelsior Cinderella, *The Penny Illustrated Paper*, 4 February 1893   39

5.1 High Class Style, Edward Scott, *Dancing as an Art and Pastime*, 1892   52

5.2 Waltzers and Waltzing, *Illustrated London News*, 1 January 1880   53

6.1 The Floral Quadrille, *The Penny Illustrated Paper*, 23 December 1893   61

6.2 What Our Waltzing Is Coming To, *Punch*, 29 January 1876   68

7.1 Learning the *Valse à Trois Temps* (Louis D'Egville) *The Tatler*, 18 January 1911   81

8.1 Dancing Class c. 1880 (George du Maurier)   91

9.1 Preparing for the King's Courts, *The Tatler*, 18 January 1911   100

10.1 Pupil Demonstrating Skirt Dance Position (Scott, *Dancing as an Art and Pastime*, 1892)   113

12.1 Alarming Scarcity, *Punch*, 11 July 1874   132

13.1 The Poetry of Motion, *Punch*, 17 February 1909   145

14.1 Society Tango, Belle Harding and partner   158

15.1 The Latest Fashion: "Pour Passer le Temps", *The Sphere*, 11 October 1913   164

15.2 Ballroom Dancing, Murray's Club   168

16.1 Reclining Nut, *Punch*, 18 March 1914   172

16.2 Time, Gentlemen, Please, *Punch*, 9 April 1913   179

17.1 Maurice and Leonora Hughes, The Crossing Step in the Ballroom Fox-Trot, *The Dancing Times*, April 1920   191

Society Dancing

Society Dancing

Fashionable Bodies in England, 1870–1920

Theresa Jill Buckland
Professor of Performing Arts, De Montfort University, UK

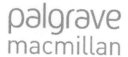

First published 2011 by
PALGRAVE MACMILLAN

Palgrave Macmillan in the UK is an imprint of Macmillan Publishers Limited, registered in England, company number 785998, of Houndmills, Basingstoke, Hampshire RG21 6XS.

Palgrave Macmillan in the US is a division of St Martin's Press LLC, 175 Fifth Avenue, New York, NY 10010.

Palgrave Macmillan is the global academic imprint of the above companies and has companies and representatives throughout the world.

Palgrave® and Macmillan® are registered trademarks in the United States, the United Kingdom, Europe and other countries.

ISBN-13: 978–0–230–27714–4   hardback

This book is printed on paper suitable for recycling and made from fully managed and sustained forest sources. Logging, pulping and manufacturing processes are expected to conform to the environmental regulations of the country of origin.

A catalogue record for this book is available from the British Library.

Library of Congress Cataloging-in-Publication Data
Buckland, Theresa.
Society dancing : fashionable bodies in England, 1870–1920 / Theresa Jill Buckland.
p. cm.
Includes index.
ISBN 978–0–230–27714–4 (hardback)
1. Dance—England—London—History—19th century. 2. Dance—England—London—History—20th century. 3. Dance—Social aspects—England—London—History—19th century. 4. Dance—Social aspects—England—London—History—20th century. 5. London (England)—Social life and customs—19th century. 6. London (England)—Social life and customs—20th century. I. Title.
GV1646.E6B84 2011
793.310904212—dc22   2011003117

Printed and bound in Great Britain by
CPI Antony Rowe, Chippenham and Eastbourne

For Tony

Acknowledgements

As a fortunate recipient of the Arts and Humanities Research Council's Research Leave scheme and Small Grants awards, I would like to thank the Council and De Montfort University for their facilitation of this research. I would also like to thank the British Academy for its support through the Small Grants scheme.

My inquiries at a number of libraries in the course of this research were always met with pleasant and helpful responses and my thanks go to staff at the British Library (St Pancras and Colindale); the Bodleian Library, Oxford; The Royal Academy of Dancing, London; The Theatre and Performance Collection, Victoria and Albert Museum, London; London Metropolitan Archives; Family Records Centre, London; City of Westminster Archives Centre; Sussex Record Office; Cambridge University Library; Jerome Robbins Dance Division, Library for the Performing Arts, New York Public Library; Brighton History Centre; Hove Library; and De Montfort University Library Services. Particular thanks go to Mollie Webb, librarian of the Imperial Society of Teachers of Dancing, London and to Sean Goddard of Sussex University Library for their support and interest in this project. Andre Gailani of Punch Cartoon Library also deserves mention for his assistance well beyond the call of duty.

I owe a great debt of gratitude to Mary Clarke and her staff of *The Dancing Times* for generously allowing me unlimited access to the first series of *The Dancing Times*. I would also like to thank the present editor, Jonathan Gray, for his help with illustrations from the journal.

Opportunities to share my findings and receive valuable advice and insight from audience members were afforded by the Centre for Dance Research, Roehampton University; Department of Dance, Film and Theatre, University of Surrey; Department of Drama, University of Exeter; Congress on Research in Dance; Society for Dance History Scholars; Dolmetsch Historical Dance Society, and my colleagues in Dance and History at De Montfort University.

For permission to reproduce copyright images, I would like to thank The Mary Evans Picture Library (cover illustration, Figures 3.1, 3.2, 8.1, 15.1); The British Library (Figures 4.1, 6.1, 7.1, 9.1) ; The Punch Cartoon Library (Figures 6.2, 12.1, 13.1, 16.1, 16.2); The Hulton Picture Library (Figure 5.2); Getty Images (Figures 14.1, 15.2) and *The Dancing Times* (Figure 17.1).

Every effort has been made to trace rights holders, but if any have been inadvertently overlooked the publishers would be pleased to make the necessary arrangements at the first opportunity.

Many friends, family, and colleagues have encouraged me throughout the long period of the book's gestation, in particular, Linda and Mick Jasper, Richard Ralph, Alexandra Carter, and my colleagues in Dance at De Montfort University. I particularly wish to express my gratitude to Margaret McGowan for her guidance.

The happy chance of sharing an office with Jane A. Adams revitalized this book project. With gentle persuasion, professional insight, and sympathetic understanding, she held my hand throughout its unfolding. My debt to her is enormous and I warmly thank her for her friendship and support.

A number of colleagues gave most generously of their time and expertise to read specific chapters and I would like especially to thank Richard Holt, Egil Bakka, and Georgiana Gore. Any errors, either of fact or interpretation, however, remain mine alone. Chris Jones has supplied counsel, a professional eye, and unwavering interest in the project, even in those early days when her valuable recommendations often fell on stony ground. In addition, my grateful thanks go to Chris for her expertise in compiling the book's index. At Palgrave Macmillan, Benjamin Doyle and Paula Kennedy have been a source of ready advice, while the team at Macmillan Publishing Solutions has patiently guided me through the production process. I wish to thank my father for valiantly reading chapters when his tastes lie more in science and engineering; and to express my appreciation to Poppy whose walks were neglected as I typed and read out huge chunks of my draft text. Above all, my most profound thanks go to my husband, Tony. He has been the best of partners dancing alongside me throughout the research and writing of this book; always ready to listen, ever willing to provide practical help, to check on my progress and to return me to the track. This book is for him.

Part I
Society Dances

1
Fashionable Bodies and Society Dancing

> Dancing always reflects the manners of the age.
>
> *The Times*, 23 May 1913

Prior to the twentieth century, dancing and deportment in European high society were designed to signal social distinction and were integral to many social rituals of royalty, aristocracy, and the upper-middle class. This was particularly so in the hierarchically conscious world of nineteenth-century England. During the late Victorian and Edwardian eras, however, this tradition irreversibly changed. The period between 1870 and 1920 saw a revolution in social dancing in Britain. The strict deportment and codified etiquette of the Victorian ball room were rejected in favour of the more relaxed and socially inclusive dance floor of the *palais de danse*. In the process, the social construction of the body changed from the 'artificial' body of the aristocratic past to that of the 'natural' body of a democratizing present.

By the end of the First World War, the European system of bodily conduct, dance, and music was moribund. Dance styles no longer arrived in London having been exclusively validated by Paris, once the undisputed centre of fashion. Instead, an increasingly mobile society looked towards New York for the latest novelties. The age of the Waltz and Quadrille had given way to ragtime dances and the Tango. Yet by the 1920s, a distinctively English style of ballroom dancing was being fashioned that was to be exported worldwide. It was to be spearheaded – not by the aristocracy who had once led dance fashion – but by the new urban middle class. If the primary aim of this book is to understand the decline of dancing as a constituent feature of royal and aristocratic socio-political life, the accompanying narrative is that of the rise of middle-class stewardship of fashion in social dancing and the ideological context for the emergence of a distinctly national style of ball room dancing.

In the Victorian and Edwardian periods, each social class of dancer may have appeared to the contemporary eye to be distinguishable from each other, the upper, middle, and lower classes of society each identifiable by their own styles and places of performance. Yet in practice, the dancing of each class was not entirely exclusive. The borders of the British class system were permeable, allowing the cultural traits of those further down the social scale to figure at times on the dance floors of their social superiors, and the traffic was never completely one way. Between the middle and upper classes, in particular, cultural assimilation of each others' mores was a characteristic of nineteenth-century England. This process was largely facilitated through individual commercial success, marriage, imitation, and increased social levelling through parliamentary means.[1]

Rather than a general survey of dancing in British society, the initial spotlight is on how dancing was fashioned and made fashionable for the cultural leaders of British society during the late Victorian and Edwardian period. Necessarily drawn into the analytical frame are the multiple and many layered issues relating to societal change that caused or resulted in the decline of dancing as a widespread and valued leisure activity and social ritual among the rich and powerful. In the process of investigating how people moved on the dance floor, I hope that new light may be shed on questions of movement and modernity that may then reverberate across other genres of dance, as well as illuminating further the social and emotional lives of those who danced.

By the 1870s, Britain was the most industrialized and powerful imperial nation in the world. Following the collapse of Paris as the leading money market after the Franco-Prussian War, London became pre-eminent as the capital of the international stock exchange. Its centrifugal force on finance had a corresponding impact on the social and cultural life of the nation and empire, as well as attracting international financiers to the rapidly expanding city (Harris, 1994). Set in motion too during this decade were a number of democratizing political transformations such as the Education Act, and civil service reforms of 1870, and the Factory Act of 1874. Such developments were to facilitate opportunities for participation in gentrified and other leisure activities further down the social scale and to assist in developing a newly moneyed urban upper-middle class whose understanding that they were living in a *modern* age became ever more conscious and articulated.

The period leading up to the First World War has been characterized by social, political, and dance historians alike as one of unprecedented change, and is often construed as a crucible of modernity whose brew of social and cultural novelties would create a turbulent impact across most aspects of life in Britain.[2] Certainly, transformations in cultural leadership and preferred movement codes from 1870 to 1920 coincide with shifting attitudes towards embodied concepts of masculinity, femininity, race, and class. If the 50 years before the First World War saw rapid change, they also witnessed deep-seated, often less vociferously articulated continuities. The beginning of the period did not herald the dawn of a new dance age: rather, it bore witness to continuing lament that the fashionable dance repertoire was stale, the conventions in the ball room ossified and largely unattractive to the younger generation. If the late Victorian ball room appeared as an outmoded and unnecessary social duty to many of its contemporaries, underneath its seemingly unchanging surface pulled many cross currents that often arose in what were regarded by the mainstream of fashionable society as cultural backwaters. In bringing some of this flotsam and jetsam to the surface of late Victorian and Edwardian dance culture, I hope to throw light on often complex and interrelated factors that are each deserving of more sustained treatment in separate study. When examining a large tract of time and the historical processes that play across it, the historian needs to give credence to the ongoing dynamic between individual effort and event, and to the less immediately visible but deeply shaping currents of longer-term factors, such as demographic change, ideological formation, and societal structure.

The focus of attention here is on those pre-First World War decades at the end of which a decisive transformation in social dancing had occurred. The manifestations of social dancing had shifted from the world of the Victorians to that of modern Britain. Dancing was no longer tied to the seasonal patterns and social segregation that had earlier distinguished the British people at play. Any attempt to comprehend that transition must necessarily engage with the wider historical debate. Late twentieth-century historians have often refuted the earlier argument of sudden rupture in favour of an analysis that interprets the various social, economic, and political developments as the inevitable advance of the intertwined processes of late capitalism and modernization.[3]

If, following the tenets of cultural history, cultural practices are inextricably linked to the domains of the social, economic, and political, then there should be a clear correspondence between social dancing and this wider evolutionary, historical context.[4] Such steady progress, however, cannot be traced in the history of social dancing in Britain; much less can its opposite – the thesis that the First World War was the primary agent in generating changes in the ball room – be upheld. The history of social dancing in late Victorian and Edwardian Britain is one neither of slow evolution nor radical change; it is altogether more complex, the sources often paradoxical and elusive.

A more illuminating interpretive framework than that of contrasting alternatives is offered by the historian Jose Harris whose characterization of the period as 'immensely varied, contradictory, and fissiparous' and in which 'social norms and expectations were widely varying' (1994, pp. 2, 3) accords with the diverse and often challenging sources that underpin this present study. Below the seemingly intractable class structure of Victorian Britain and its associated culture, divergent dance practices often broke through the class barriers, contesting accepted norms, sometimes disappearing altogether, then re-emerging much later in new guises.

Social distinction and fashionable dancing

In examining fashionable dancing in England during that period, I concentrate on activities that centred on London, then the largest and premier trading capital of the world.[5] Its cultural leaders were the cream of the English aristocracy, envied at home and abroad as 'the most wealthy, the most powerful, and the most glamorous people' (Cannadine, 1996, p. 2) in Britain. Their cosmopolitan lifestyle of conspicuous consumption was displayed at its most extravagant in the frequent and large private balls that were hosted and attended every year by this socially restricted community, during the ritual known as the London Season.[6] This customary gathering in the capital took place in the spring and early summer months, and was a vibrant, if conservative, institution from the eighteenth century that brought together the most important families of the land. These privileged few, together with the royal family at the helm, constituted the social group known as Society, a group set apart in the writing of outsiders by the convention of the initial capital 'S'. Additionally referred to as polite society, the best circles, the Upper Ten Thousand, or simply the Upper Ten, Society was an exclusive group that sought to preserve its social, political, and economic superiority during the rapidly changing world of Queen Victoria's final years. As one of their many pleasures, dancing was almost a daily occurrence during the London Season and was frequently practised during the rest of the year as a pastime and social ceremony.

The 1870s proved to be 'the last decade of apparently undisputed patrician pre-eminence' (Cannadine, 1996, p. 8), a time when this small social elite that owned and led an extensive empire, might claim adherence from the majority of its members to the corporeal rituals established over several centuries. During the following decades, retention of Society's once seemingly stable and royally focused culture became a pressing concern for its members, many of whom perceived a number of threats to their lifestyle. Among their anxieties were the declining wealth of many aristocratic families, the seeming invasion of the newly moneyed into their once select community, the increasing profile of rich trans-Atlantic brides among their noble kin, and popular antagonism towards the profligacy of the alternative court of the Prince of Wales.[7] In the 1870s, the political, economic, and cultural ascendancy of the aristocracy and its social rituals appeared unassailable. By the 1920s, the prominence of the Season and the significance of its dance events were in marked decline. Increasing social mobility, changes in patterns of public and private entertainment, shifts in gender expectations, and the popular influence of African-American music and dance, were contributory factors whose deleterious impact on this ritualized behaviour were consolidated by the First World War. The Upper Ten Thousand who had once determined fashion in Britain and its empire now followed rather than led. After the First World War, Society's continuity as 'high society', much expanded in numbers and diluted in aristocratic composition, was testimony to the progressive diminution in power of its royal leaders. With Society's slow decline went the significance of dancing in socio-political life in Britain.

For much of the nineteenth century, Society had been a dominant force, composed of a tightly knit social elite, loosely based on aristocratic kinship, and whose borders were keenly patrolled by its womenfolk. Beyond the criterion of family, further measures of fashion and etiquette operated as visible and interconnected means of regulating entry to Society's ranks. The Upper Ten's display of fashionable attire as a measure of social station looked to Paris, a city that from the seventeenth century had governed tastes in dancing and in dress, particularly for aristocratic women. The Upper Ten's rehearsal of etiquette was based upon conservative modes of conduct that hailed from the British royal court and which were sanctioned in practices outside its inner circles by courtiers and followers-on.

Exemplary performances of fashion and etiquette reached their apogee in the London ball room. There, the gathering of Society, which was reckoned to represent the most civilized and cultured element of British society at large was 'on its very best behaviour', its activities 'regulated according to the strict code of good breeding.'[8] In the 1870s, London Society ball rooms were filled with well-bred dancers of aristocratic lineage, their highly codified and well-ordered deportment and dancing the result of years of training by dancing teachers. The role of Society's dancing and deportment instructors was to fashion bodies that instantly stood out as belonging to a superior station in life, moving according to a genteel code, and dancing the latest dances. Both Society men and women were schooled early in this bodily distinction, though, as objects of wealth and grace, women more than men were subject to the dictates of being fashioned and fashionable.[9] For the young Society woman, the London Season was a time and space for expensive and tasteful exhibition; it constituted an important rite of passage, the numerous balls and private dances of the Season providing her with a means of entering the marriage market. London Society and its balls maintained the world depicted in the early nineteenth-century novels of Jane Austen, where marriage gave women status and men a male heir to their estates.

In spite of the stratified class structure, movement up the social scale in Victorian Britain was a genuine possibility for those with money, connections, and a willingness to abide by the conventions of Society's formalized world. As the nation's prosperity and empire grew during the nineteenth century, so too did the number of families desirous to become ennobled and to live the lifestyle of Society. For those who were neither to the manor nor manner born, there existed an industry of professional help on Society behaviour, ranging from texts such as etiquette books and advice columns in Society journals to more personalized support from tailors, dressmakers, and dancing teachers.[10] Even if ardent followers of the latest fashions of Society had no real hope of acceptance as one of their number, the cult of gentility functioned as a means to set off the socially aspirational from those immediately below on the social ladder. English society was notoriously finicky in its recognition of social gradation through outward appearance: nuances of dress, deportment, dancing, and speech were readily grasped and interpreted as evidence of social station, though such seemingly superficial signs were perceived as ridiculously snobbish by foreigners and those of a higher moral persuasion.

In line with these values of social distinction, the overall dance culture of late-nineteenth and early-twentieth century Britain strongly echoed Victorian preoccupation with individual and family status. Where and when people danced underlined the strict hierarchy of the nation's social, political, and economic order. Geography, personnel, venue, and frequency of dancing combined to articulate a deeply class-conscious society. Income and social standing determined the resources of time and space available, and it was this combination, rather than any exclusive repertoire, that identified the dancing behaviour of the different social strata. Princes and princesses, lords and ladies, the families of rich businessmen, bankers, lowly clerks, and tradespeople may have whirled round the ball room in the ubiquitous Waltz and also stepped through the figures of the long-established Quadrilles – but very rarely did they do so together: the recreational dance culture of late Victorian and Edwardian Britain was a socially segregated and hierarchical affair.[11]

Each of the three main social groups in Britain that possessed the time and money to enjoy dancing on a regular basis followed a different temporal and spatial pattern in which to pursue their dancing. At the top end of the social scale stood Society, its inner sanctum made up of the monarchy and the landed classes who consisted of the hereditary peerage and the non-titular gentry. Together, this small but powerful group enjoyed a nomadic pattern of dancing that coincided with annual moves from their country estates to London in spring until early summer for the Season, to Scotland for shooting game towards early autumn, and to fashionable resorts in continental Europe in the early winter. Its members could indulge in dancing with comparative frequency, as the constraints of shop or office hours did not impose on their daily existence; for the 'idle rich', unemployment was both the privilege and the distinguishing feature of true gentility.

Below them in the social scale came those who needed to work: the wealthy businessmen and professionals such as financiers, lawyers, and well-to-do doctors whose income allowed them to attend more upmarket public venues for dancing. They aimed to follow the accessible fashions of their social superiors, but were necessarily more limited in their geographical mobility and in their spare time. The upper-middle class's dancing season usually lasted from October to early June and centred on cities. As their numbers and affluence grew, the upper-middle class began to extend their dancing activities into the established leisure resorts of the aristocracy, aping their culture as far as their means might allow. During annual summer holidays, particularly from the 1890s onwards, the richer fashionable families might be discovered dancing at smart seaside resorts on the continent, often in the casinos and large hotels on the northern coast of France.

Such luxurious locations for dancing were not, however, within reach of the more middling sort of British society. Their summertime dancing was more likely to take place during the week or a few days away in the British coastal resorts. During the winter and early summer months, this class of people, typically composed of the owners of small businesses, the better-paid clerks, managers, and more upmarket shop assistants, attended public dances in their local towns and cities, often on a monthly or weekly basis. Their access to recreational dancing profited greatly from the reduction in working hours, increases in their pay, and better, more affordable public transport.[12]

For those on the edges of Society, a coveted invitation to one of the numerous dance events held out the possibility of social advancement and acceptance within the fold of power and influence. Acting as a yardstick against which the rest of the British population might measure their own social position, Society was the source of much envious and sometimes censorious interest among the middle classes. For the socially ambitious, keen to stand alongside Britain's ruling aristocracy, whether through marriage or money, or both, the acquisition of patrician habits of dance and deportment was considered highly desirable. Such bodily expertise was profiled each year during the ruling class's residence in London; but access to the balls and dances enjoyed by royalty, aristocracy, and the favoured few was strictly limited. Invitations were only issued within its tight community: the influential elite held its dances behind closed doors for most of Victoria's long reign.

Social dancing in polite society required a basic level of competence in a limited number of dance forms that had been in vogue for the greater part of the century: among them, predominantly, the Waltz and the Quadrille.[13] Both dance forms continued to be performed at state balls until after the First World War. The Waltz, the favourite dance of many in late Victorian society, was the most prominent example of the category of round dances, so called because dancing couples turned on their own axis as they circled the ball room. The Quadrille, on the other hand, was classified as a square or set dance, designated by the spatial formation taken by the set of four couples, or sometimes multiples of four, whose evolutions were traced largely within and around the enclosed square they defined on the dance floor.

Contrasting in number of dances, use of space, and musical rhythm, the Waltz and Quadrille offered complementary physical and social sensations. The Waltz attracted by its promise of a tight embrace and feeling of headiness as the man and woman whirled together, lost in a world of their own; the Quadrille, more sedate in its choreography, facilitated social and physical interaction among several couples at a time. Each dance form fulfilled the distinct needs of Victorian high society: the Quadrille, successor to the eighteenth-century Minuet, was the perfect vehicle for the ceremonial opening of a ball; the Waltz, symbol of romance, proffered the ideal overture to courtship. Towards the end of the nineteenth century, when alternative arenas emerged for young Society men and women to socialize and when royal and aristocratic power was under attack, the function of these dance forms became destabilized, helping to open the door more widely to a vigorous new repertoire that deliberately flouted the restricted decorum of the late Victorian and Edwardian Society ball room.

In their place, just before the accession of George V, came a seeming cacophony of dances from America that was thought by many contemporaries to represent the end of the civilized world. To others, this invasion was a welcome breath of new life that signalled the potential of genuine challenge to outdated Victorian convention. 'On or about December 1910,' Virginia Woolf (1924) famously declared, 'human character changed.' The precise dating of this change was, as Woolf acknowledged, quite arbitrary. Nonetheless she pinpointed a moment when social and artistic experience joined to articulate a decisive shift away from the long prevailing world view that became characterized as Victorian. Woolf's statement, later interpreted as identifying the birth of literary modernism, found resonance with forms of visual arts, music, fashion, and theatre that began to appear in the second decade of the twentieth century. At the same time, that discernible rupture with the past became visible in social dancing.

This visibility was more pronounced not only on account of the greater numbers now entering Society, but also because of the related necessity to seek more and larger venues for its dance events. Society's dancing now took place in public rather than in private. The ball rooms of London's mansions were eschewed in favour of the opulent, less personal, ball rooms of London's new hotels, notably the Savoy and the Ritz. For the older Society hostesses, control of the dance and music repertoire was easier to maintain at events held in the home, but the new hotels and restaurants were the scene of the latest fashions in entertainment and were popular with the young. In 1910, onlookers in London's fashionable ball rooms witnessed a succession of new dances accompanied by music with distinctive rhythmic features that were drawn from African America. This was a repertoire that introduced fresh cultural features that were to lay stylistic foundations for the rest of the century. Its syncopated rhythms and opportunity for individualistic expression appeared to stand in direct opposition to the melodic flow and co-operative choreography of the Victorian ball room. Rags, Trots, and Tangos were poised to replace the Waltz, Polka, and Quadrille. The rhythmic traditions of Africa were to engage with the melodic dominance of Europe in a manner never previously sustained in mainstream popular culture.

By the end of that second decade, Britain had turned her face firmly towards America. It was from across the Atlantic that future choreographic innovations in popular dance were to arrive over the next decades – even if a vague desire that they travel the traditional route of cultural authentication, via the hotspots of France, was to endure a few more years. Ultimately, however, France's centuries-old pre-eminence in dictating guidelines for fashioning the bodies of Europe's ruling elite was at an end. The performance of political and economic power through embodied cultural capital belonged to a vanished world, its remnants occasionally to be recalled in the lingering ceremony of British Society's debutantes and their presentation at court.

The rest of British society had, however, moved on; far more exciting and accessible was what American music and dance had to offer, and a young generation recovering from the devastation of the war eagerly seized the vitality of the newly powerful nation's cultural offerings. Among the influential British bourgeoisie, however, deeply impregnated by the genteel values of their country's former rulers, total renunciation of the aristocratic bodily codes to which they had aspired and sought to copy, and moreover which appeared to them and to many in the world to constitute the essence of English identity was not to be effected so rapidly. In the new style of English ball room dancing that emerged in the 1920s, the cultural hegemony of the aristocracy remained clearly visible.

2
Fashioning Dance Histories

> In this age, where the current of research is set so
> strongly in the careful seeking after truth, the claims of
> the dance on the consideration of the British reading
> world must rest on a broader basis than that of being
> a mere amusement for the light-minded.
>
> Lilly Grove, Dancing, 1895, pp. 1–2

The sphere of the social has largely remained the Cinderella of dance studies. It has frequently been assigned to the categories of folk dance or historical dance, neither of which has featured strongly in Anglo-American academic dance discourse.[1] The reasons for this neglect can partially be located in conceptualizations of dancing that draw upon European distinctions between the realms of the artistic and the social, the professional and the amateur; distinctions that can be traced back at least to the European courts of the late seventeenth century when dancing as a theatricalized form, performed by professionals, emerged as a discrete practice.[2]

Until the early twentieth century, traffic in dance practices across stage and salon, between the professional and the amateur, remained fluid. Hard and fast division of classification and practice between the social and the theatrical is a later phenomenon. The flow across stage, salon and indeed street is rarely reflected in twentieth-century mainstream dance scholarship. Instead, a hierarchical dichotomy between dance as art and dance as a social or ritual practice became cemented in Euro-American literature.[3]

A driving factor in shaping this critical discourse was the legitimation of dance as one of the liberal arts by writers and artists, both within and outside the theatrical profession. Exploration of this significant shift in the perception, conceptualization, and valorization of dance practices awaits more detailed and sustained analysis. Suffice it to state here that theatre or concert dance in the early twentieth century came to be viewed as a higher, more evolved form, with its roots in the comparatively simple social or ritual forms of dance. In a trajectory that closely parallels the development of musicology as an academic discipline, much of the foundational literature on dance as an academic discipline has emphasized the repertoire, performers, and creators of European art dance: those dance practices that were regarded as communal and popular, supposedly requiring little specialist knowledge to perform, have been discounted as subjects too familiar, ephemeral, and lacking in complexity to merit attention.[4] The popular has been equated with the trivial, a topic deemed suitable for coffee table books, and for general histories aimed at amateur enthusiasts and the interested general public.[5]

A more conducive climate for the academic treatment of social dancing emerged in the closing decades of the twentieth century when wide changes in perspective swept across theoretical and methodological paradigms in the arts and humanities. Of particular significance for dance history were three interrelated developments: the so-called cultural turn, a new interest in the hermeneutics of the human body; and postmodernist approaches to the past.

For much of the twentieth century, interpretation and classification in dance historiography were mediated through a nineteenth-century evolutionist and racist framework. Dance anthropologist Joann W Kealiinohomoku published the first sustained critique of this pervasive perspective in 1970, but the implications of her exposé largely went unheeded until the 'cultural turn' of the 1980s when literary and cultural studies furnished the principal filter into dance scholarship.[6] The intellectual expansion generated by the influence of the 'cultural turn' encouraged a move away from analysis of the dance art work per se to its wider context of cultural signification. Cultural relativity – once the shibboleth of anthropologists – helped to expand the research agenda, including that of dance historiography. Occurring alongside feminist discourse in the arts, and critical analyses of the operations of power and the politics of culture, such approaches stimulated scholarly interest in dance forms and practices that had previously been positioned as 'other' to the mainstream of Eurocentric theatre and concert dance. Postcolonial theory gave greater voice to the dancing of the subaltern, the values of cultural diversity being claimed for practices once summarily dismissed as inferior or ignored.

A second development that has influenced studies of dance history was the late twentieth-century explosion of literature on 'the body' across academia. This had the salutary effect of promoting dance as a subject of potential scrutiny for scholars outside the discipline of dance studies. While it was theoretically enriching, much of this non-specialist literature tended to avoid close attention to the dance itself. Instead, arguments of cultural representation, located in the static rather than the moving body, dominated new research, even sometimes within the discipline of dance. As many dance specialists observed, the baby seemed to have danced out of the bath water. From the mid 1990s, some scholars influenced by variants of phenomenology, feminism, and critical reflexivity in the social sciences, returned dancing to a more central position.[7] In this fresh departure, issues of structure and history remained in the shadows as new considerations of embodied agency took precedence.

In the first decade of the twenty-first century, such theoretical and methodological strategies were applied to a number of studies in dance history, their authors highlighting personal sensory perceptions in their construction of forgotten dance forms. Problems exist with such approaches, not the least of which is the often unrecognized projection of a universalist notion of the body.[8] Caution needs to be exercised if excessive reliance is placed on the heuristic potential of embodiment. Anachronistic interpretations may result if the dance historian trusts the embodied experience of the present uncritically. Historians of dance, in company with other researchers of the past, experience difficulties of interpretation when seeking to recreate a 'world that we have lost'. But they have an added problem of seeking corporeal understanding, full access to which is inevitably limited by the irretrievable and multifaceted nature of the physical conditions that fashioned the once moving bodies of the past. This unavoidable sense of the remoteness of history, particularly in its quotidian and largely unarticulated sense, brings me to touch briefly on the third consideration of influence in late-twentieth century dance historiography – the impact of postmodernism.

The ferocious controversy surrounding postmodernist approaches in the discipline of history during the 1980s and 1990s has lessened in the early twenty-first century. The debate over extreme positions of absolute cultural relativism and the rejection of historicity, versus unwavering belief in source-based criticism and the limits of theory have left their traces in dance historiography. In light of dance's comparatively late acceptance as an academic discipline, it can be argued that the timing of postmodernism's impact on its fledging status was not altogether beneficial. The more extreme instances of postmodernist research tended to detract attention away from the value of archival immersion in dance history, resulting in restriction of the potential of inquiry.[9] Nonetheless the craft of dance historiography has gained expansively and intensively from these interrelated challenges to established historical inquiry. The various debates and new formulations and procedures have facilitated more nuanced, reflexive studies in which the corporeality of dancing engages with theoretical substance and that in the more rigorous research, avoids the sins of reductionism and presentism.

Traces of dancing

Historians have frequently noted the comparative number and variety of historical sources on the educated, leisured, and powerful. In a literate society, this volume typically increases in modern times, providing a plethora of archival data that renders full cognizance and use of every source impossible. Like many historians, the interpreter of dance may narrow this often almost overwhelming abundance by choosing to focus on an individual, a key event, a short-lived institution, or a very limited temporal range.[10] To address cultural change and continuity, however, demands examination of a wider span of years and limitation of the sources to hand. Data on social dancing in late Victorian and Edwardian England is richly diverse, embracing dance manuals, etiquette books, journals and newspapers, paintings, photographs, sheet music, diaries, local histories, autobiographies, and fiction. Added to this, census returns, wills, street directories, and birth, marriage and death certificates supply further vital information of a socio-economic nature. Analysis of these latter sources can offer a keener understanding of the relative social status of individuals and of the demographic changes that affected the profession of dance pedagogy.

In the second half of the nineteenth century, Britain had a well-established press industry including daily, weekly, and monthly newspapers that catered for different strata in society. There was also an expanding number of specialist-interest journals published for the professions, trades, and leisure interests of an increasingly literate nation.[11] For the upper echelons *The Times* had become the newspaper of choice, serving as the main organ of social communication for the ever growing Upper Ten, whose membership had long outgrown the logistics of oral communication. *The Times* was the principal contemporary source for notice of royal engagements and forthcoming Society balls; it listed the diary of the London Season, ran occasional reports on noteworthy dances of the social elite, especially if they were attended by royalty, foreign dignitaries, and high-ranking nobility, and carried columns of adver-tisements which included those of the dancing teachers who sought an aristocratic and well-heeled clientele. The *Daily Telegraph* and the *Morning Post* offered similar material, with more localized newspapers such as the *Hampstead and High Express* and the *Kensington News* serving the needs of the well-to-do middle classes resident in these mainly bourgeois inhab-ited districts of London.

By far the most extensive coverage of social dancing for the upper-class participant can be found in the journals produced for Society women. Prominent examples of the period are *The Queen* and *The Ladies Pictorial* which supplied high-class tasteful gossip on the royal and aris-tocratic celebrities of the day, ran regular articles on the various leisure pursuits of the rich and noble, listed recent and forthcoming balls and prominent dances, and detailed the latest Parisian fashions.[12] Similar, if not quite so exclusive, provision was repeated in daily and weekly newspapers, their proprietors capitalizing on the growing female mar-ket. Women's columns dedicated to female interests began to occur later in the century, covering information on fashionable dress and etiquette. Articles on how to give dances and how to behave at them fed the mid-dle classes' appetite for the life to which they aspired. Regular notes and queries in the press addressed the niceties of social decorum, assuaging the anxieties of the newcomer or the socially aspirational, desperate to be accepted as a *bona fide* member of the Victorian 'in-crowd'.

The articles are rarely signed – a feature typical of Victorian writing, and common in the correspondence columns, even into the initial decades of the twentieth century. This preservation of anonymity often proved as frustrating to contemporaries as to present-day historians. A notorious example is the letter to the *Times* in 1913 which was signed 'A Peeress'. The author's identity was never revealed, but her comments on the mores in the ballroom of the day sparked a controversy that reverber-ated among upper- and middle-class devotees and opponents of dancing (see Chapter 16). It also, as in the 1897 letter to the press on a similar theme by the Countess of Ancaster, provided easy, topical copy.[13] Care needs to be exercised in granting full credence to some press items, particularly reports on ragtime and jazz dancing that were undoubtedly exaggerated for sensationalist impact. This type of coverage does have the advantage, however, of providing some insight into what newspa-pers believed to be of potential interest to readers, especially regarding the latest 'smart' or 'modern' vogue.

A further characteristic of the Victorian press was the habitual re-publication of articles and notices from other contemporary sources.

Not only did the practice fill pages, but it also cascaded information down the social scale, informing the middle classes how the 'best circles' conducted their cultural affairs. When specialist publications on dancing appeared in the early 1890s, items from Society journals and newspapers provoked discussion in editorials and correspondence columns on the state of affairs in the ball room and the potential future of dance pedagogy. They also re-reprinted historical snippets and translations of recent publications on dance theory and history.

The earliest of these professional dance journals in Britain was the London dancing master Robert Crompton's *Dancing*. Beginning in June 1891, this was published each month during the urban dancing season that ran from September to June until its last issue in May 1893. Contemporaries of *Dancing* were the first series of the *Dancing Times*, produced by another London dancing master, Edward Humphrey from 1894 until around 1902, and *The Ball Room*, established in 1894 and distributed by dancing teachers Mr and Mrs Johnson. Sadly, no copies of the latter survive, as a result of the bombing of the British Museum's holdings during the Second World War, a fate that was shared by many contemporaneous books and ephemera relating to dance.[14]

Prescriptive manuals, etiquette books and technical aides created by dancing teachers provide some of the most extensive but often frustrating sources of information. Frequently, these publications contain unacknowledged material recycled from earlier studies, especially from eighteenth-century texts.[15] There also exist problems in identifying some authors with certainty. Many of the etiquette books were ghost written, their author known only as that elusive figure, 'a member of the aristocracy' or 'a gentleman of title'. In a number of cases these anonymous guides were written by those able to observe the aristocracy, often close servants, and so familiar with Society etiquette. By the end of the nineteenth century, named members of Society were authoring guides, notable examples being Lady Violet Greville or, a little further down the social hierarchy, the Honourable Mrs Armytage, expert on court ritual.[16]

Dancing teachers who catered for the middle class, such as London-based Miss Leonora Geary and Mr and Mrs Henderson, regularly compiled *aide memoires* to the ball room, continuing the earlier practice of dance pedagogues. This literature was typically in the form of a pocket book that might be taken to a dance event for easy reference. Although these books were principally for their pupils, the teachers sought wider sales through newspaper advertisements that gave notice of their classes and copies of their ballroom guides in exchange for postage stamps.[17] As access to literacy and leisure time improved further down the social scale, the expanding publishing trade took on more of this production of cheap dance manuals. The notorious activity of 'puffing', hyping recent publications, had declined by the later nineteenth century; nonetheless, the promotional literature cannot be taken at face value, and even internal documentation, such as the number of editions, needs to be treated with caution. What is clearly discernible, however, is a growing movement towards scholarly engagement with the theory and history of dance, as evidenced in the publications by Edward Scott (1899) and Lilly Grove (1895) and later by Reginald St. Johnston (1906), J. E. Crawford Flitch (1912), Cecil Sharp (1907–13), and Ethel Urlin [1914].

Some ball room guides contained musical examples, often as a further promotional device by the publisher. Sheet music production grew exponentially throughout the Victorian period, as the middle classes entertained one another at home, with parlour songs, piano music, and dancing. The adaptation of popular melodies from the stage, both opera and musical theatre, increased from the 1880s, and the imagery of their cover sheets is sometimes illustrative of the dancing, the musical instrumentation, and social context.[18] How this music was played in practice is less easy to decipher. A number of dancing teachers maintained the eighteenth-century tradition of musical composition, playing the violin, and leading dance bands themselves.[19] Their publications are of especial interest, although again, clues to the realization of these musical notations are limited.

Representations of dancing in action can be culled from the numerous visual images in the satirical weekly magazine *Punch*. This famous journal published an extensive array of cartoons depicting social *faux pas* in the ballroom. Allowing for the necessary exaggeration to achieve comic effect, many of the cartoons nonetheless illustrate social foibles on or around the dance floor that can be verified from other sources. Two further factors in the evaluation need to be borne in mind: first, many *Punch* artists of the period followed a lithographic tradition of historical verisimilitude; and second, a number of *Punch* illustrators themselves frequented ball rooms.[20] Throughout this 50 year period, the *Illustrated London News* portrayed dance events attended by the social elite, whereas the cheaper *Penny Illustrated Paper* favoured dancing assemblies of the middle class at the Holborn Town Hall, Portman Rooms, and Cavendish Rooms in central London. Depicting dancing at opposite ends of the social scale, *Punch* illustrator Phil May (1864–1903) was well known for his sympathetic illustrations of the London working class. His work in the *Daily Graphic* provides valuable comparative material on dance styles.

Dancing was also a subject for Victorian painters, notably James Tissot whose scenes of fashionable London in the 1870s did not escape contemporary criticism for their suggestion of illicit or compromised relations; more frequently, the ball room became a trope for the minor genre of paintings that looked to illustrate eighteenth-century manners as models of civilization (see Chapters 6 and 10). These imaginary ball room scenes from the previous century are symptomatic of the Victorian fascination with the past. Numerous photographs of people in fancy dress at the hugely popular costume balls also bear testimony to the obsession with dressing up in historical clothes. Most of the images, as for example in the well-documented Duchess of Devonshire's Ball in 1897 (see Murphy, 1985) are portraits of the great and the good in their chosen attire, playing at being exotic or reincarnations of their ancestors. More commercially focused and indicative of movement are the picture cards of theatre stars and female entertainers taken in photography studios. These can supplement knowledge of exhibition dance genres, such as skirt dancing, which was popular on the stage and widely imitated by Society ladies and children for the entertainment of their own social circle. By the end of the first decade of the twentieth century, photography was overtaking lithographic illustrations in Society journals; photographs of stage celebrities performing dance crazes such as the Tango, Grizzly Bear, and Turkey Trot appear alongside publicity images of famous exhibition ballroom dancers. Fuelling public appetite for the latest dance novelty, press photographs also helped to promote the careers of entrepreneurial dance teachers such as Belle Harding (see Chapter 14).

Access to the personal experience of the dancer is fleetingly granted in the literature of the aristocracy whose nostalgia for the leisured extravagance of Society is captured in the numerous autobiographies written after the First World War. Contemporaneous responses can be gleaned from diaries, but the more sustained considerations of dancing are recorded in the new publications geared towards the social dancer. The most focused, informed, and consistent of these is the second series of *The Dancing Times* that appeared monthly from 1910. Edited by Philip Richardson, himself a keen ballroom dancer with experience from the late 1880s, the *Dancing Times* quickly became established as the main discursive forum for ballroom dancing, a position that it continued to occupy for several decades. Richardson (1946, 1960) played a pivotal role in the promotion and institutionalization of dance teaching in Britain, and his reminiscences and narrative history remain essential reading.[21] A. H. Franks, his immediate successor as editor of the *Dancing Times* and author of *Social Dance: A Short History* (1963), builds upon

Richardson's work, although his treatment is more ambitious, both in terms of chronology and in relating dance to the wider social context. Richardson's influence is hard to sidestep when looking for alternative perspectives from the period: disagreement there undoubtedly was with respect to preferred styles of performance and constructions of historical lineage, but these voices appear muted as a result of the more limited and scattered nature of their record.[22]

3
The Seasonal Round

> To learn this social code, this unwritten body of stat-
> utes, is ... the labour of a lifetime.
> Lady Greville, *The Gentlewoman in Society*,
> 1892, p. 2

The occasions on which Society met to dance were legion, especially during the London Season, where balls and dances far outnumbered those available for dancers further down the social scale. At formal private balls, the older and married among Society danced alongside the young and unattached, but at the comparatively few public dances, all participants, regardless of age, kept to their own class, or sets of family and acquaintances. Ideally, all the guests took their turn on the dance floor, the only exceptions being the elderly infirm, the physically incapacitated, and the chaperones, whose duties forbade them from putting their own pleasure before that of their younger charges.[1]

At the more prestigious balls in the capital, dancers included members of royalty, leading politicians, and visiting foreign dignitaries. These gatherings were opportunities for extravagant displays of fashionable dress, costly jewels, and stylishly abundant floral decorations within the magnificent town houses. They were also occasions punctuated around midnight by the consumption of a handsome supper and huge quantities of champagne. The architectural splendour of the private venue, the social rank of the guests, and sheer opulence of provision acted as competitive markers of Society taste and fashion.

Society's cohesive nature was traditionally conserved by the customary practices of endogamous marriage and primogeniture. By the mid-nineteenth century, its numbers had expanded mainly as a result of improving birth and infant survival rates; through marriage with other large landowners, especially in Scotland and Ireland; and through the limited inclusion of very rich merchants who desired to adopt the status and lifestyle of the English gentry (Colley, 2005). Victorian Society perceived itself as British, although the descriptor 'English' was often used as a substitute, indicating where the hub of government and influence lay.

In the wake of the American War of Independence (1775–83) and the French Revolution (1789), the British elite had felt distinctly nervous, watching anxiously as successive revolutions overthrew royal and noble governance on the European continent. On the economic front, Britain's home-grown Industrial Revolution had also posed challenges to the existing social order: a rapidly expanding industrial and professional bourgeoisie began to seek greater access and control of the country's social and political fortunes. These threats wrought changes in Society's behaviour during the nineteenth century, and this was distinguishable in their choice of venues for dancing.

The Upper Ten withdrew from public assembly rooms and gardens to dance in one another's residences, the richer among them building grandiose ball rooms to accommodate their guests. A complete retreat was impossible, however, not least because the continued acceptance of the aristocracy's privileged position was largely dependent upon the support of those immediately outside Society's borders, and whose entrepreneurial skills and wealth helped to inject new blood into its aristocratic veins. A select number of these were invited to attend the county and charity balls that were held predominantly outside the London Season in public spaces (see Chapter 4).

Although by the late nineteenth century, the class structure in Britain had become notably rigid, it remained possible to travel up the social chain through three principal means. These well-trodden pathways comprised the possession of extraordinary wealth, a strategic marriage, or the bestowal of land and honours from the Crown. Whereas Society counted these pathways as legitimate, they were also potentially open to the social climber, the philanderer, or, most heinous of sins in genteel society, the 'vulgar'.

Married women from the most important families in the land assiduously patrolled Society's borders, determining the acceptance or rejection of new people and new cultural practices. This matriarchal domination of a highly nuanced code of both ethical and aesthetic conduct helped to distinguish and replicate Society in its own image (Davidoff, 1973). Only through birth not purchase into an authentic ancient lineage, they argued, could the true gentleman and lady be fashioned and uniquely embody the singular conduct and good taste that were the hallmarks of true nobility.

In spite of its accelerating numbers from the 1870s onwards, Society remained dominated by fewer than 30 families who were excessively wealthy and close to the Royal family (Cannadine, 1996). It was these who mounted the most expensive and ornate dance events, comparable to and at times surpassing the magnificence of the state balls. Their lifestyle was resourced from land and property rents, plus exploitation of natural resources on their estate. Profiting from and contributing to Britain's development into the world's leading economic power, they had helped to secure London's authority. No wonder that their sayings and doings were instant and constant topics of press reports.

By the last third of the nineteenth century, their extreme wealth was being matched, even challenged, by the rise of the new breed of plutocrats, as Britain's imperial conquests and control created new wealth among the landless classes. A very small number of these were incorporated into the innermost sanctum of Society, most notably into the Marlborough Set around the Prince of Wales. This composite of royalty, aristocrats of ancient English lineage, Jewish bankers, and South African millionaires, sprinkled with a few theatre celebrities possessing wit and beauty, was notorious for its hedonistic and expensive lifestyle. Following the Prince's example, established aristocracy began to welcome more of the newly moneyed, the foreign, and the famous into their fashionable lifestyle.[2]

The balls and dances of the London Season

Society's pleasures during the London Season took place within a narrowly circumscribed geographical space. The estates of royalty and aristocracy may have been spread across the British Isles, but the principal rites of the ruling class took place within less than a few square miles in the West End of London. Centred on Mayfair and St James with Buckingham Palace and Marlborough House as a royal focus, the space of London's *beau monde* was bounded to the north by Oxford Street, to the south by the House of Commons, to the west from Alexandra Gate to the South Kensington Museum, and to the east by Regent Street. Here, a passer-by might catch a glimpse of Society in full evening dress moving from carriage to door to attend a magnificent ball.

The most prestigious and select of all the balls were those given by the Royal family. Such grand occasions were employed to receive visiting dignitaries and to celebrate state and family anniversaries, birthdays,

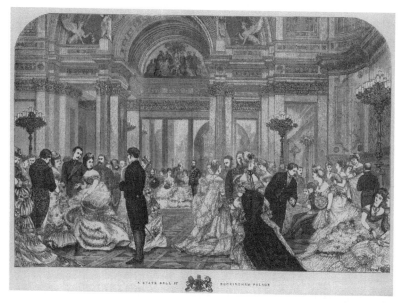

Figure 3.1   A State Ball at Buckingham Palace, 1870

and weddings. Following the death of Victoria's Consort, Prince Albert, in 1861, the heir to the throne, Edward, Prince of Wales, and his wife, Alexandra, hosted the state balls held at Buckingham Palace, deputizing for the now-reclusive Queen. Victoria retained control of the list of invitees; all names of potential guests being passed to her for approval by the Lord Chamberlain who also acted as master of ceremonies at the state balls. In the 1880s, upwards of a thousand invitations at a time were issued, challenging the capacity of the royal ball room (see Figure 3.1).

There were, however, a number of other royally patronized balls that the favoured might attend, not least of which were those hosted by Edward and Alexandra at their own residence of Marlborough House. Similar in size and splendour were the balls held at Stafford House (now Lancaster House) Cleveland Row, a magnificent London palace, which Queen Victoria had reputedly viewed with more than a tinge of jealousy (Chancellor, 1908). As Society had relocated its pleasures into the private sphere, there had been a spate of extensions and improvements to old houses and a commissioning of new building. Several of the most magnificent London residences lined the edges of Hyde Park and St James's Park, the address of Park Lane Mayfair being 'synonymous with worldly riches and fashionable life' (Chancellor, 1908, p. 249).

Many London palaces housed massive ball rooms or art galleries that doubled as spaces for dancing. Especially desirable was an imposing staircase, from which individuals might see and be seen. The slow-moving line of bejewelled and decorated Society guests, waiting to shake hands with the ball hostess positioned at the top of the staircase, provided ample time for observation and display.[3]

A large ball room and impressive staircase were not the only architectural necessities for a Royal or aristocratic ball; further extensive space was required for separate cloakrooms for men and women, the latter containing, as well as general attendants, maids who were on standby to repair torn gowns. Other expected facilities were a refreshment room, separate from that of the supper room, which was usually located downstairs; a card room for the men whose active dancing days were over or whose interests did not extend to frequent waltzing; and small alcoves or balconies where the elderly or those wishing to converse might sit in comfort. At the more exceptional events, marquees and covered walkways were erected in the gardens, which were also transformed into magical spaces, with coloured lights and Chinese lanterns hung from trees and bushes.

It remained easier for those with vast country estates and armies of servants to mount the grander affairs. Given the sheer scale of some of these balls, it is not surprising that the Countess of Ancaster (1895) observed that the stately homes of England with their even larger premises were perhaps better suited to entertaining than the London houses. But the centre for extravagant show remained the capital, and the Countess favourably compared the comfort and splendour of London balls in the 1890s with those of her youth. Produce from Duchy land and greenhouses, together with wine and champagne from aristocratic cellars, was supplied for the enormous feasts that constituted the obligatory formal cold supper. Huge quantities of exotic flowers, with their overpowering scent, and large tropical palms were transported from estate gardens and hothouses to decorate the London palaces in the latest fashion. The expensive and safer electric lighting had replaced the earlier century's candles and gaslight, adding an extra brilliance to the jewels of the women in their low-cut ball gowns. On the walls of the ball rooms of the great London palaces, Grosvenor House, Stafford House, Montagu House, Wimborne House and Dorchester House, portraits of their owners' aristocratic ancestors and valuable paintings by the great masters looked down on the resplendent dancers. Sometimes the appearance of the dancing figures bore an uncanny resemblance to those depicted in the paintings: on very grand occasions, royals and aristocrats enjoyed fancy dress and historical costume balls, finding a ready source of inspiration for their costumes among their own art treasures. When the Prince and Princess of Wales hosted a grand fancy dress ball in the season of 1874, the *Times* (23 July) pronounced approvingly that 'the pride of our people requires that there should be a well-ordered magnificence in the lives of their Princes, and certainly his Royal Highness the Prince of Wales proved himself last night well descended from Kings whose Courts have never been wanting in splendour'. In contrast to these ostentatious events, Society's private dances differed from the ball by the numbers invited, the copiousness of house decoration, and the fulsomeness of the supper. Especially popular outside of the London Season were the afternoon dances known as 'small and earlies' that ran from four to seven o'clock in the evening. Whereas a ball typically attracted upward of three hundred guests, a dance was designed to accommodate between 80 and 200 guests. Unlike the fashionable large string orchestra of Coote and Tinney and the Hungarian Band employed for royal balls, a small group of two or three musicians (piano, cornet, and sometimes violin) was thought adequate to accompany the many dances that typically took place in a converted drawing room. For even smaller and more impromptu affairs, a single pianist was common, etiquette books recommending, however, the hire of a professional rather than obliging a female guest to play.

Afternoon dances were also popular with the less wealthy as they did not require costly floral decorations and extra lighting. They also saved money on refreshments: rather than the expensive champagne, wine, cold meats, salads, and deserts that were *de rigueur* at a ball, tea, coffee, soft drinks, sandwiches, and cakes were the typical fare. Instead of the expense of evening dress, the dress code was comparatively relaxed: the women wore light summer gowns or day dresses with walking shoes and bonnets, and the men attended in morning coats.

For those families thrown upon their own resources at home, turning a drawing room into a miniature ball room, however, was not a task to be undertaken lightly. The drawing room had to be cleared of furniture, the carpet rolled up, and in some cases windows removed from their frames to ensure sufficient ventilation when the room was crowded. Blocks of sculptured ice were another device to cool down the guests on crowded, hot summer evenings.

The majority of dances during the London Season took place in comparatively small drawing rooms where the grandeur of the affluent ball-givers' marble dance floors gave way to the modern utility of wooden parquet. More usually, Society members as well as middle-class families stretched a special fine cloth, called drugget, over the drawing room carpet to provide a smooth surface for dancing, a practice that gave rise to the popular name, 'carpet dance'. On occasions when the carpet was lifted, the wooden floor revealed underneath often had to be sanded down and polished to produce a suitable dance surface. Preparations involved considerable extra work for the servants, and manuals recommended that to cut down on the expense of hiring more help, the family's children could be enlisted to help polish the floor by sliding up and down with dusters attached to their feet.

Afternoon dances were not only popular as home entertainment. The economies of scale were preferred by many military and navy men, who threw balls and dances to return the hospitality of their host settlement. High-ranking members of the country's armed forces, traditionally composed of the second sons of the aristocracy, belonged to Society, but that did not guarantee disposable income. There were many officers, especially with families to raise, who did not have surplus money to foot the bills of a large scale ball. An afternoon dance, often known as a 'barrack' or 'garrison' dance, avoided extra expense as the event could be housed in the garrison, the music supplied by their own band, the food by their mess, and the dancing space decorated with the regimental silver.

Ball room etiquette in Society

Invitations to balls and dances in private residences were issued by the senior female member of the household, normally the wife; in the case of a bachelor or widower, this task would be undertaken by a sister or daughter. As well as respectable family and friends, the list for invitation might also include individuals who were in a position to advance the careers or marriage prospects of sons and daughters. The first arrivals at a typical London Society ball were usually the young women, accompanied by their chaperones, and eager to dance away the evening with many prospective suitors. Dressed in their evening finery of low-cut long dresses, their arms bare, necks and hair adorned with jewellery, they remained around the edges of the room, until invited to dance, an arrangement resulting in the popular soubriquet 'wallflower'. Other mixed parties began to arrive after dinner or the theatre, before the anticipated influx of young men, many of whom had lingered in the all-male ambience of their London club appeared towards midnight.

Such dilatory attendance by the young men was not countenanced in the grander balls where everyone gathered before the arrival of the royal party. The royals were always greeted at the door by the host and hostess at a London ball, the dancing commencing only after the royal procession to the ball room. Every Society ball was opened by a Quadrille, sometimes of eight or sixteen couples, in which the hostess led with the gentleman of highest rank. Only then did more general dancing follow, but royal etiquette demanded that other guests vacate the floor when the royal party danced.

Within all Society ball rooms, conduct was strictly regulated by an etiquette that had evolved to protect the interests of the wider social group (St. George, 1993), adherence to which, according to commentators, reflected British society at its best. A large Society ball was in essence a microcosm of Victorian society, the manifestation of civilization in its highest social guise. The expected performance of duty by every individual present at the ball perfectly illustrates the Victorian philosopher John Stuart Mill's (1869, p. 124) observation that

> the English are farther from a state of nature than any other modern people. They are, more than any other people, a product of civilization and discipline. England is the country in which social discipline has most succeeded, not so much in conquering, as in suppressing, whatever is liable to conflict with it. The English, more than any other people, not only act but feel according to rule.

Though on a less humanitarian scale than Mills's opinions on female emancipation with which this quotation is concerned, the proliferation of etiquette books and dancing masters' manuals underlines the obsession with form that characterized high Society and its imitators. At a Society ball, guests were never free to select their preferred partner for each dance, but instead were expected to subjugate their own feelings to ensure the pleasure of everyone present. The aim was for everyone to co-operate to create a perfect community

> where all are for the time as one large and happy family, of which each member is solicitous for the welfare of his fellows, and careful that nothing is said or done that may destroy the harmony of the evening.
>
> (Scott, [1885], p. 7)

Within this larger family of Society, it was considered 'bad form' for young women to refuse an invitation to dance if they were free to do so; for married men to dance with their own wives; and for men and women to dance with one another more than twice within an evening.

The man's special privilege to invite a woman to dance came with various restrictions, the most prominent of which was that he might not approach a woman unknown to him without first seeking a formal introduction from the dance's hostess, or daughters, known family, or a mutual friend. Decorum forbade any woman to ask a man to dance and many debutantes, overlooked at their first appearance in London, spent many an hour in the cloakroom pretending that their dress needed to be repaired, rather than face the misery and ignominy of sitting out yet another dance. To ease such situations, to improve the young women's chances of finding a matrimonial match, married women, especially those acting in the capacity of chaperones, were expected to abstain from dancing. The chaperone's duties were to ensure that their charges circulated among the company, neither spending too much time dancing and talking with any one man, nor cultivating romance with those deemed socially undesirable. Society ladies had their own vernacular for such individuals: a rich bachelor of good family and personal reputation was judged a 'parti', his opposite a 'detrimental'.[4]

To assist memory, programmes with pencils attached enabled guests to note the names of accepted partners alongside the 18 or 20 dances that typically made up an evening. The dance that occurred just before supper had special significance. Unless a gentleman needed to honour a prior commitment, such as looking after an older female relative, he was obliged to accompany his partner from this dance to supper. There, he was to attend to her needs throughout, and, unless she was contracted to another partner for the first dance after supper, he was bound to escort her back to the ball room. Manipulation of the card's record to accommodate preferred later arriving partners or failure to honour the written contract threatened an individual's reputation. The conduct of the flirtatious Gwendolen Harleth in George Eliot's *Daniel Deronda* (1876) was undoubtedly not unknown in reality: she plays with the conventions of being invited to dance in her quest to make herself distinctive in the ball room and ultimately dance with the most high-ranking eligible individual present (see Figure 3.2).

By the 1880s, if not earlier in some quarters, programmes had gone out of fashion in London Society, except where they were produced as mementos of some exceptional costume or state ball. They remained in regular use at semi-public or masked balls, and in the shires where there was more mingling between the classes. Society claimed that programmes were not necessary in the Season where guests were restricted to their own social milieu. No doubt, though, the declining use of programmes at Society dances was cemented by the increased tendency

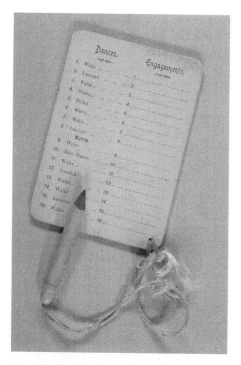

Figure 3.2   Dance Card, Late Nineteenth Century

in the London Season for parties to move from dance to dance in the course of an evening, in search of friends or, as often as not, a more fashionable gathering: given the changing composition at a dance, there was no guarantee that the promised partner was even still in the building when the band struck up the agreed Waltz or Quadrille.[5]

Hosting a glittering ball was an excellent strategy for a relative newcomer to become better connected, but relied upon the co-operation and favours from those already within Society's fold. A sympathetic female friend higher up the social scale issued invitations to her own more select circle of acquaintances, adding her name on the card alongside that of the hostess. Depending on the venue and rumoured hospitality of the event, eminently fashionable members of Society, keen to enjoy the lavish pleasures that extreme wealth could provide, might be enticed to the *parvenu's* ball. According to the custom of reciprocal hospitality, this new family might then succeed in having their names added to the guest lists of polite society; providing, of course that, as new acquaintances, they were sufficiently wealthy and respectable in their conduct. In this 'gift exchange', the ball guest list operated as a form of cultural capital, highly coveted by members of the *nouveaux riches* and, for the poorer members of the aristocracy, a useful disposable asset. A classic fictional example occurs in Anthony Trollope's novel, *The Way We Live Now*, published in 1875. Financial swindler Augustus Melmotte's acceptance into Society reaches a summit when, in the company of high-ranking members of the aristocracy the Prince makes his appearance at the ball and partners Melmotte's daughter in a Quadrille. This episode, as elsewhere in the novel, nicely satirizes the infiltration of Society by the newly rich in search of influence. It is also testimony to the social charisma still exercised by the old landed aristocracy, in spite of their dwindling finances and lessening political power.

This social and often financial transaction between old and new Society attracted more than fictional comment. In 1889, the satirist and Society entertainer George Grossmith was asked by the *Pall Mall Gazette* how it was that new arrivals in London of 'colonial swells' and 'American millionaires' were soon described in the Society press as the hosts of 'smart and splendid' dances:

> Oh! it is quite simple if you have lots of money and a friend at court who knows everybody. The friend asks the guests, the friend turns the house into a huge and odiferous bower of exotics, the friend weaves the garlands of roses which trail so gloriously up the staircases, the friend sees the mountains of ice which rear their glittering crests up to the ceiling, and the hostess at the top of the staircase doesn't know a dozen out of the thousand who fill her rooms, and is perfectly happy.[6]

Grossmith's observation chimes with the activities of minor courtier Percy Armytage (1927) whose expertise and enjoyment in planning state balls and similar royal ceremonies on behalf of the Lord Chamberlain led to a professional career in ball organization, much to the chagrin of his aristocratic family. He was by no means alone in profiting from the sale of his cultural knowledge and social connections. Many of his class and influence were forced by economic necessity to follow a similar, if less glamorous, path.

In contrast to the top 30 families, many aristocrats in the late nineteenth century struggled to maintain the houses and lifestyle that the London Season demanded. As a consequence of geography and geology, not all noble families had been able to profit from the Industrial Revolution. By the 1880s, declining land rents, coupled with falling wheat prices, prompted many to reduce their expenditure and to seek fresh sources of revenue so that they might continue to participate in the most significant events of the London Season (Cannadine, 1996).

The need to maintain a profile in the London Season was high. Frequent appearances at the balls and dances of a Season, fashionably dressed and *au fait* with the latest ways of dancing and behaving, might consolidate the social reputation of a wife and, by extension, the family; or, more strategically, visibility at the balls and dances might secure a daughter's marriage to a wealthier, hopefully titled, son of Society. Fathers and guardians met huge bills from the dressmakers, especially those of the favoured fashion house of Worth in Paris, from dancing teachers, shoemakers, hairdressers, florists, and household servants – as well as maintaining a carriage to transport the family to balls and other events, for Society members never travelled by public transport. Furthermore, it was necessary to return hospitality and provide a platform to display daughters by hosting a ball or dance.

As landed families sought to reduce the costs of the Season, they began either to rent or sell their London houses to richer members of their class or to the *nouveaux riches*. By the 1890s, it was quite usual for less wealthy aristocrats to take reduced lodgings at a reasonably smart address in London's West End and then to rent a spacious house in a prestigious quarter for their own ball or dance (Armytage, 1927). More servants and waiters were then hired specifically for the event, thus cutting down on domestic expenditure for the majority of the Season. Other income for the impoverished gentry, it was commonly whispered, was procured by the sale of expertise in etiquette and influence. Such transactions met the demand for social advancement from indigenous social climbers and, increasingly, from rich foreign bankers, diamond millionaires, and other wealthy industrialists from the United States, South Africa, and other British colonies.

The high profile marriages of American heiresses, such as the Jerome Sisters and Consuelo Vanderbilt, who had married into the upper echelons of British society, attracted similar seekers of aristocratic title from across the Atlantic.[7] The British assumed from such illustrious matches that all American visitors to Society were wealthy suitors who were prepared to exchange new wealth for old world status. This rumoured practice of 'cash for Society membership ' was satirised by Canadian Sara Jeanette Duncan, whose eponymous heroine, in the semi-autobiographical *An American Girl in London* of 1891, travels through the London Season's calendar, oblivious to her hosts' wrongly placed zeal to secure her as a rich wife for one of their low-ranking bachelors. The Society dance that Duncan describes is delivered with the sharp, independent eye of a documentary journalist, whose freer-mannered upbringing across the Atlantic affords her a view of the famed reserve and seemingly joyless experience of the upper-class English at play. In the rented house used for Lady Powderby's dance,

> the ball upstairs was going on with the same profound and deter-mined action as the ball downstairs.... the same universal look of concentration, the same firm or nervous intention of properly dis-charging the responsibilities of the evening and the numbers on the programme, on the face of the sweet, fresh *débutante*, steadily getting pinker, as the middle-aged military man, dancing like a disjointed fort-rule; of the stout old lady in crimson silk, very low in the neck who sat against the wall. The popular theory seemed to be that the dancing was something to be Done – the consideration of enjoyment brought it to a lower plane.
>
> (pp. 175–7)

It is this contrast between the attitudes of the old and new worlds that reverberates to more poignant significance in the novels of American-born authors Henry James and Edith Wharton.

In the late nineteenth century, Americans may have appeared brash and even barbaric in their manners to many in Old World society (see Pells, 1997), but their new country's growing economic and political con-fidence would impact strongly on European culture, particularly dance, in the forthcoming century. For the moment, English Society maintained the upper hand in accommodating the culture of the rising numbers of American visitors and residents in London. Wherever it could, Society clung to its belief that potential marital partners and guests should evince not only wealth but also breeding. Lacking a monarchy and aris-tocracy, the United States' nearest equivalent to Society was the famed Four Hundred, the oldest and richest of the original settler families who formed America's social elite; it was this fashionable, rich, and similarly exclusive community who possessed the potential to marry into Society. In spite of gossip to the contrary, money was not the sole ambition of the British aristocracy: true to their traditional values, and wherever and for as long as possible, Society continued to privilege class, especially if accompanied by good looks and wit, over the single criterion of cash.

4
Public Spaces

> Balls this year as a means of paying hospitalities
> and welcoming one's friends will be largely given at
> numberless semi-public halls or other central places of
> entertainment.
>
> *The Lady's Pictorial*, 24 December 1887, p. 653

Outside the London Season, Society attended the public, or perhaps more
accurately semi-public, county and charity balls held in the shires. These
long-established dance events reflected the highly stratified nature of
British society more generally. The annual county ball brought together
the families of the leading aristocracy, lesser gentry, and professional
classes, usually in the assembly rooms of the county towns, in a performance of the social order. Its metropolitan equivalent was the Inhabitants'
Ball or Mayor's Ball at which the upper-middle class, in their role as local
politicians and powerful employers, outnumbered the county aristocracy
and gentry.

Within the traditional county ball room, the classes remained strictly
segregated: the most important space was occupied by the highest ranking at the top of the room, notably the aristocracy who played a crucial
role in county politics and economics; the lowest members, though
never less than the richest and most influential among the county,
danced at the bottom. Even in the early 1870s, some county balls maintained the practice of dividing the room by a cord suspended across the
space, though this was rare. Instead, in the later Victorian era, this class
apartheid relied upon the stewards to monitor the conduct of their own
social stratum, and upon the self-imposed restraint of the guests to keep
to their proper set. Tickets for the public dances of Society were typically acquired by requesting vouchers from the ladies' committee which

were then presented to the male stewards or honorary secretary for each party of guests to attend. This method of advance social sanction was carried out by committees and stewards drawn from each level of the society expected to attend. Tickets were never on open sale or available at the door, and this system of subscription by voucher and ticket preserved the select nature of the gathering.[1]

The typical county ball repertoire largely mirrored that seen in London ball rooms, although it might include a few more of the vigorous dances such as Polkas and Galops, as well as the less fashionable country dances, particular favourites being *The Triumph* and *Sir Roger de Coverley*. The private Hunt Balls of the winter, attended by the fox-hunting community, shared a similar repertoire, providing another opportunity for large house parties from nearby stately homes to continue their social networking and entertainment in the quieter months of the seasonal round.

At public charity balls, Society shared philanthropic concerns with the great and good of the locality. Expected to bestow largesse upon the less socially fortunate, the ladies of the aristocracy and gentry acted as patronesses, granting use of their names 'to lend éclat and prestige' (A Member of the Aristocracy, 1888, p. 219) making financial donations to the charity, or providing game from the country shoots for the ball supper. Where it was a charity close to the family's interest, or more cynically where there was the promise of a favourite band and fashionable friends, the patronesses were likely to appear, their local celebrity status promoting the sale of tickets. The chief organizers worked hard to secure the patronage and attendance of as many fashionable ladies, or even royalty, as possible: indeed, the lure of celebrity worked among Society just as much as among the bourgeoisie.

Nowhere was this more apparent than in the most famous of Victorian charity balls, the Royal Caledonian. Unusually among charity dances, it took place during the London Season when so many of the British aristocracy with estates in Scotland gathered in sufficient force to merit holding such an event in the capital. It was organized on an annual basis at Willis's Rooms and later at the Whitehall Rooms, Hotel Métropole, and attracted not only the richest Scottish aristocrats but also royal patronage in raising funds for the Royal Caledonian Asylum and the Royal Scottish Hospital. Established by the Duke and Duchess of Atholl in the 1840s, the Caledonian Ball became a highpoint of the Season's calendar. Its Scottish theme was reflected in several ways: the Highland dress worn by some of its guests; the opening Highland Quadrille in which the organizing patronesses danced, dressed in white, each with tartan sashes of their Scottish clan, and the repertoire that, unusually for the London Season, included the energetic reels and strathspeys deemed native to Scotland. Fancy or Highland dress was compulsory and Society ladies were keen to be asked to attend rehearsals to prepare, if not for the Highland Quadrille, then for the other of the two main ceremonial Quadrilles which, during the 1870s, was often a Poudré Quadrille, performed in eighteenth-century costumes, the dancers appearing with powdered faces and wigs.[2]

These semi-public balls were housed in large, often multi-purpose rooms, used for concerts, lectures, and exhibitions as well as dances; but their amenities rarely equalled the comfort, glamour, and quality of Society's town residences. Whereas Society danced on the continent in magnificent hotels, London lacked comparable premises for entertaining. Earlier in the century, British aristocrat men on business visits had both dined and slept overnight at their London clubs, or if travelling with their families rented rooms at respectable addresses. Following London's growth into a premier financial capital, large hotels were constructed, commencing with the large railway hotels that housed the rising numbers of itinerant businessmen from provincial towns and cities. By the 1880s, London was attracting thousands of visitors from the United States, the European continent and the colonies, counting foreign royalty and aristocracy, and visiting magnates and their families.[3]

At first, Society shied away from the new hotels, until theatre impresario Richard D'Oyly Carte successfully courted the Prince of Wales and the Marlborough Set to his new luxurious hotel, the Savoy (Clayton, 2005). Opened in 1889 on the Strand, close to the heart of theatre land, the Savoy housed a spacious and opulently decorated ball room, a gourmet restaurant, and the comfort of accommodation facilities equivalent to those on the continent, and the east coast of the United States. The Savoy's success in attracting the rich, the royal, and the famous was followed by further new and modified building of the Hotel Cecil (1886), Claridges (1894), the Cadogan (1895), the Ritz (1908), and the Waldorf Hilton (1908), the hotel interior designs closely modelled on the royal and aristocratic palaces. Sealed by royal approval, these new luxury hotels began to be regularly patronized by Society for their dances: by the 1900s, Society ball hostesses increasingly eschewed the disorder and discomfort of crowded home dances for the relative ease of hiring the new large and comfortable public spaces.

Dancing further down the social scale

Until the later nineteenth century, the upper-middle class aimed to emulate Society's rites of passage by holding private dances for their marriageable offspring in the somewhat cramped confines of their own town houses. Mothers, aunts, and elder sisters, living on the edge of London's West End, in districts such as Kensington and Bayswater, sought advice from Society journal reports and the frequent editions of *Manners and Tone of Good Society* and *Party-Giving on Every Scale* on how best to adapt their more spatially limited accommodation, but still be up to date and socially correct.

With the vast population expansion in the capital, there was increasing pressure to move outwards to more space in the new villas of suburban Hampstead, Richmond, and Blackheath, or to rent the new apartments, closer to the city centre in Kensington and Chelsea. Neither style of abode was advantageous as a private dance venue: the first was located too distant from the city to attract a fashionable crowd, and the second was too small, and subject to complaints of noise from neighbouring flat-dwellers.[4] Moreover, there was a growing shortage of servants in the capital, as many lower down the social scale chose to reject a lifetime of drudgery in domestic service, opting for better career opportunities in office work or department stores.

These factors, together with the dreaded upheaval that hosting a dance at home entailed, caused the middle class to lead the exodus from the domestic arena in search of new public venues for dancing. Coupled with these physical drivers were the growing leisure interests of a more affluent and time-richer stratum of society, with access to good transport connections, and to new restaurants and galleries, in a city that by the 1890s was undergoing a cultural renaissance (Clayton, 2005).

Dances were held in conjunction with a variety of social gatherings among the upper-middle class: an annual ball to bring together the members of a professional group; a monthly, fortnightly or weekly dance for those in a special interest society; or a series of subscription dances to support one of the many charity fund-raising events. The model of the Upper Ten's events was assiduously followed by this class: 'everything is as correct as in the highest strata of society, from the faultless evening dress of the men to the robes à queue of the damsel and young matrons.'[5]

The more upmarket of these dance events were held at St James's Hall in Regent Street, the long-established Willis's Rooms (formerly known as Almack's Assembly Rooms), the Portman Rooms in Baker Street, and the recently built Princes Hall on Piccadilly, opened by the Prince and Princess of Wales. At this latter venue, a long-running subscription series, known as the Prince's Cinderellas, was launched in 1885, to raise funds for the Chelsea Hospital for Women. Earlier in the decade another subscription series of Cinderella dances was established at the new Italianate-designed Kensington Town Hall. Catering for City men, lawyers, barristers, and their families, this series was primarily for pleasurable rather than charitable purposes and continued on an annual basis until at least the First World War. Not surprisingly, the 'Cinderella' style of event was popular with the middle class in general for, as the name suggests, the dances concluded before midnight, enabling dancers to attend them mid week and still get up for work in the morning (see Figure 4.1).

At the Portman Rooms, 'acknowledged to be the most magnificent rooms in London', a comparable winter series of dances was the Excelsior Cinderellas organized by dancing master Robert Crompton during the 1890s.[6] Annual subscription to these cost one guinea, but tickets to a single dance, applied for in advance, could be obtained for two shillings. In the 1890s, the Portman Rooms were the scene of several charity balls, such as those run by the Primrose League; for institutional

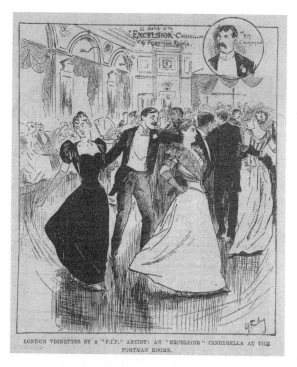

LONDON VIGNETTES BY A "P.I.P." ARTIST: AN "EXCELSIOR" CINDERELLA AT THE PORTMAN ROOMS.

Figure 4.1   Excelsior Cinderella, *The Penny Illustrated Paper*, 4 February 1893

organizations, such as Masonic Lodges, and Hospitals; for societies of professionals such as the Chemists' Assistants' Association; for military regiments; and for an increasing number of special interest societies, ranging from lawn tennis, cricket, football, swimming, and golf clubs, to musical and dramatic groups such as the Haydn Musical Society.[7] Dancing was a valued way of raising money for public concerns, and a healthy means of socializing for people whose urban, office-based work life was increasingly sedentary.

For the middle class, an invitation to a high-status public ball, held at one of the new large town halls in London's districts, or more impressively at the older, more central Mansion House or Guild Hall for example, signalled social acceptance, and the opportunity to mingle, in however a restricted manner, with the great and the good. Local government officials and businessmen viewed large dances as a means of bringing together representatives and their families from various trades and businesses, to cement loyalties; it was an excellent opportunity for the organizers to exercise largesse, in the urban equivalent of the tenants' and servants' balls hosted by the aristocracy on their country estates.

Social pretensions, often coupled with ignorance of how events were conducted among the higher reaches of society were a frequent subject for ironic comment in the press and in novels. George Grossmith created one of English literature's most endearing if risible characters of this ilk in Mr Pooter, the hero of *The Diary of a Nobody* (1892). Pooter, a lower-middle-class clerk and suburban dweller, is thrilled and filled with self-importance at being invited, together with his wife, to attend a function at London's Mansion House. His gradual deflation with regard to the actual social significance of the event and his own class position culminates at the ball, as his pride literally takes a fall, when he and his wife end up in a heap on the highly polished floor. Pooter's narration of the ball and the events leading up to it ironically exposes his own social ignorance. The fall was the result of his refusal to follow his wife's sound advice to scratch or wet the under soles of his new boots; instead, he complains, in a mistakenly superior manner, that the highly polished floor should have been covered by a drugget – a strategy, known to the less socially naïve, as being more appropriate to a small carpet dance than to a ball at the Mansion House. Having greeted the invitation's arrival as public affirmation of his family's upward trajectory, Pooter is further irritated at the ball to find himself in the company of the local ironmonger, for, as a City office worker, he regards himself as superior to tradesmen. The episode is an excellent depiction of the nuances of English social status in operation at a ball; social distinction is not only performed and recognized *between* classes, but, *within* a class, most notably that of the rising middle strata, for whom the cult of gentility exercised such a significant means of social evaluation.[8]

The location of social dancing beyond Society's preferred public venues was closely mapped onto a finely graded scale of social position and pretension. Less grand than the Portman Rooms, but still appealing to a 'higher class' clientele, were the Cavendish Rooms, near Oxford Street in central London, which belonged to dancing master Edward Humphrey. These upgraded premises were a timely and lucrative response to the growing need to house 'Private Parties, At Homes, Private Theatricals, and other Social Festivities'. An advertisement for hire of the facilities offered:

> 12 rooms, consisting of a larger and smaller ball-room, capable of accommodating 150 dancers; these rooms are beautifully decorated, lighted by electricity; and the specially-laid floors, exquisitely polished, are acknowledged to be the best in London for dancing purposes. There is a large refreshment or supper room, which seats comfortably 160 persons. Several delightful lobbies, ante-rooms, card-rooms, &c., are arranged and furnished for the "sit-out," so essential for the modern ball-room; though with such a perfect floor, and the capital band attached to the premises, conducted by an eminent composer, the "sitters-out" are few and far between. The ladies' and gentlemens' retiring rooms are perfect of their kind. The whole suite of rooms are thoroughly ventilated, and are always cool and refreshing.[9]

For the price of one guinea, dancers could attend more than one hundred dances a year ranging across 'petits bals', special evening dress parties, costume dances, and summer dress parties.

Humphrey's seasonal round of classes and dances was a more extensive and diverse provision than that offered by most urban dancing teachers, whose operations were typically accommodated in less comfortable and fashionable spaces. At their own dancing academies, urban dancing teachers organized weekly dances, known as assemblies, for pupils to practise their steps and to socialize with one another. Larger venues, however, were needed in *fin-de-siècle* London to accommodate the growing army of clerks in the City and shop assistants in the new London department stores, who, with more time and higher wages than that previously available to the lower-middle class, sought to indulge their enthusiasm for dancing on a regular basis.

The most well known of these large public dances were the 'select assemblies', held every Saturday and Monday from 8 p.m. to 11:30 p.m.

at the Holborn Town Hall. Under the guidance of dancing master H. R. Johnson these popular dances were attended by around 200 to 300 mostly young people, dressed in their Sunday best, rather than in the expensive evening dress of Society and the upper bourgeoisie. For special occasions, the more successful dancing masters organized balls at grander venues, where they often requested evening or fancy dress to be worn. Francis Piaggio, for example, organized themed balls at the Portman Rooms, his annual St Patrick's nights attracting around a thousand people.[10]

From the closing decades of the nineteenth century, subscription dances held by cricket, football, golf, and lawn tennis clubs provided opportunity for the well heeled to dance more frequently. Out in the suburbs or wider afield in the provinces, these mainly annual series of dances were normally held during the winter months. They were often organized not by dancing teachers but by a committee made up of members from the club. This was typically led by a secretary, who saw to the printing of the circular and tickets, hired a hall, contracted caterers, secured a band, and sometimes acted as M.C. Tickets were predominantly sold to family and friends of the committee members who hoped for a small profit to maintain their sports facilities. In 1910, an article in the *Dancing Times* on how to run a subscription dance suggested that a dance for about 100 people would need to price tickets at seven shillings and sixpence each. A number of these dance series were long lived: the Vesta Rowing Club, for example, celebrated its 26th season of subscription dances in 1911 at the Empress Rooms.[11]

A more popular form of subscription series in the leafy suburbs of London was the 'Picnic' dance, the oldest being the Hampstead Picnic Dances established in the early 1890s at Hampstead Drill Hall. Typically each committee member was charged to bring a party of around ten people, evenly balanced by gender. As the name suggests, picnic dances were distinguished from other subscription dances by their catering arrangements. Whereas a subscription dance usually offered a hot supper, drinks, and often soup for all dancers at the end of the evening, at a picnic dance, each committee member was responsible for organizing the food for her or his own party. Picnic dances were especially popular in the suburbs, where parties often divided the task of bringing sandwiches, cakes, claret, and soft drinks between them rather than running to the expense of outside caterers.

For the growing number of keen upper-middle class dancers, the subscription series organized by sports clubs and the like could not always guarantee sufficient expert dancers or a gendered balance of partners.

The directive behind subscription dances was shifting away from dances as occasions to raise funds or to socialize towards dances as occasions in their own right: dancing was fast becoming the primary motivation for the event rather than the adjunct of an existing social institution. This transition from dance's earlier epiphenomenal character to a central *raison d'etre* marks the dance practices of a modern urban society. Here was a dancing community rather than a community that dances; and this phenomenon was to become further distinguished among some dancing communities in the early twentieth century by an increasing focus upon one specific dance form.

Whereas devotees of dancing among the upper bourgeoisie paid attention to stylish dancing, most public dance occasions were not organized for the display and nurturing of dance technique. For many in Society, appearance at a fashionable event for social purposes far outweighed any desire to strive for terpsichorean perfection. By the 1890s, a sprinkling of Society might be seen at public dances, as a new generation, eager to participate in the booming nightlife of *fin-de-siècle* London, tested the tired conventions of their parents and grandparents. The most notorious of these public dances was the Covent Garden Costume Ball. Inspired by the masked balls at the Paris Opera, theatre proprietor Sir Augustus Harris instituted the annual series during the winter of 1892, predominantly as an income generator during the dark months of the theatre. These costume balls attracted hundreds of revellers, sometimes, indeed, thousands on opening and closing nights of the series.[12]

On payment of a guinea, a member of the public could dance in the huge auditorium; or for half a crown, watch the dancers below from the amphitheatre, and admire the themed sets – perhaps the Riviera of the Mediterranean or London By Night. Restrictions on public gatherings had obviously eased by the 1890s, as on arrival at the door, dancers could also hire a mask and a domino – the long black-hooded cloak worn at Venetian carnivals that completely shrouded the identity of the wearer. Masked balls had only recently returned to favour in England. Earlier in the century, the upper class's fear of social disorder had precluded disguise at any but the smallest of private dances. The Covent Garden Costume Balls were testimony to a loosening of such social controls; it should be noted, however, that there was always a police presence outside the theatre, and entry was restricted to those able to afford evening or fancy dress. Elaborate and novel costumes were encouraged by expensive prizes, such as a Steinway piano, a fashionable dress from the House of Worth, or diamond jewellery, awarded around four o'clock in the morning.[13] Given such hours, the event was not frequented by the middle class of regular working hours and good reputation but, as journalist Robert Machray (1902, p. 145) characterized them, the fast set:

> officers of the army, men from the Stock Exchange, actors, journalists, betting men, men about town, young 'bloods,' and hosts of men who can only be described as nondescripts, except that they are all bent on seeing life and resolved to quaff the purple cup to the dregs.

The female clientele were not wives or chaperoned young women, but the 'Half-World' of mistresses and well-dressed prostitutes that frequented the vicinity of theatre land. Less than a decade later, however, young Society women were among the winners of the fancy dress competitions, indicating a growth in respectability of the Covent Garden Balls, and, more especially, the changing expectations of young women, the more headstrong of whom were keen to equal their brothers in enjoying a hedonistic lifestyle (see Chapter 10). For the fast set, predominantly made up of young and unattached men who were not so tightly tied to the constraints of respectability as their sisters, the hedonistic world of Bohemia, with its late night parties, often beckoned. In pursuit of the novel and slightly risqué, leisured youth, or *jeunesse dorée* (gilded youth) as Society journalists referred to them, sought out new sensations, approving the latest in theatre and music, and taking advantage of the social licence prompted by fancy dress.

Fashionable for the very rich throughout the later nineteenth century, fancy dress and historical costume balls extended their appeal to the leisured and wealthy (Holt, [1879]), especially in the early twentieth century as a means of raising money for charity. Unlike the famous Duchess of Devonshire's Ball held to celebrate Queen Victoria's Diamond Jubilee in 1897 (Murphy, 1985) which was a strictly private and exclusive affair among royals and aristocrats, the themed balls in the vibrant early years of George V's reign crammed together the fashionable, aristocratic, fast, and artistic sets. In addition to the Savoy Hotel, the Royal Albert Hall was a popular venue for these private charity balls, making full use of its capacious ballroom which, at 16,000 square feet, was reckoned in 1913 to be the largest in the world.[14]

Typically attracting around 4000 people, these events were equalled in popularity, and to some extent patronized by many of the same clientele, by the fancy dress balls of the Chelsea Arts Club and the Three Arts Club. Entry was still controlled by a subscription system for tickets, but barriers were beginning to become more relaxed at these semi-public affairs. Whereas Society had earlier frowned on social mixing between their own kind and the world of artists, the once discrete communities of Mayfair and Bohemia, as these social rather than geographical spheres were respectively known, now met openly to socialize through dressing up, drinking, and dancing until dawn.[15] Chaperones were out of fashion in this carnivalesque atmosphere, where the focus was on fun not duty. Little attention was paid to the niceties of dance technique in such venues: firstly, dancing tended to take second place to the main activities of drinking, eating, and horseplay, or else the space was so crowded that it proved impossible to dance. During much of the evening, the crush was so great that dancing was often reduced to walking to the Waltzes and Two-Steps played by the regularly hired Corelli Windeatt's band. The only serious opportunity to demonstrate any traditional dancing expertise occurred in the opening ceremonial Quadrilles, performed by family, friends, and favourites of the committee members, and choreographed by leading Society dancing teachers, notably Louis D'Egville: to shine in such a spectacle, still required the services of an eminent dancing master familiar with instructing royalty and nobility.

5
Late Victorian Repertoire

> [T]here is no reason why ball-room dancing of today
> should not be as characteristic of refinement, grace, and
> elegance, as those more stately and intricate dances of
> our forefathers.
>
> Robert Crompton, *Theory and Practice of Modern*
> *Dancing*, [1891], p. 16

Towards the end of the nineteenth century, there is increasing evidence of public discussion and complaint about dancing standards and changing behaviour in the Society ball room. Care, however, needs to be exercised in interpreting such records. Dancing teachers had a long tradition of bewailing falling standards and opportunities for recording complaint expanded in the late nineteenth century with the exponential growth of the publishing trade. Nonetheless the number and nature of contributions to the debate indicate quite decisively that real changes were occurring that moved beyond the carping of specialist interest groups and further than those prone to disaffected comparison with times past on the basis of fanciful nostalgia. By examining manuals such as Edward Scott's *Dancing As It Should Be* (1887a), taking note of the admonitions made in prescriptive texts, and listening to the voices of those within Society, a picture of changing social and aesthetic norms within the late Victorian ball room clearly emerges.

From formality to jollity: The Quadrille

The First Set of Quadrilles had replaced the Minuet in the early nineteenth century as the opening ceremonial dance of the court ball (Richardson, 1960). Typically performed by four couples arranged as the sides of a

square, its numbers of couples could be doubled, tripled, or even quad-
rupled on all sides to accommodate larger numbers, as at an important
state ball. Often noted on the programme simply as the First Set, or
Quadrille, the dance received its name by virtue of being the first set of
Quadrilles to be performed in fashionable London society.[1] Its structure
of five figures, *Le Pantalon, L'Été, La Poule, La Trenise* (or sometimes *La
Pastorale*), and *Le Grand Rond*, each of contrasting rhythmic or general
musical character, mostly in 4/4 and occasional 6/8 time, provided the
model for later compositions. There were hundreds of sets of Quadrille
figures invented and published by dancing teachers during the century,
but the First Set continued to dominate. As dancing master Robert
Crompton observed ([1891] p. 60):

> In different parts of the country, as well as amongst different grades
> of society, slight variations of the figures may occasionally be met
> with, but no embarrassment will occur to a dancer, who is thor-
> oughly familiar with the orthodox rules for performing the several
> movements used in Set Dances generally.

A set of four couples required around 25 square yards in which to
dance, with a distance of ten to twelve feet between opposite couples,
to enable them to travel smoothly in relation to the musical phrasing
(Humphrey, [1874]; Scott, 1892). Characteristically, the leading first
or top couple, who stood with their backs to the musicians, began the
Quadrille, and danced with the couple facing opposite them, known as
the second or bottom couple. The figure was then initiated in turn by
each of the four couples around the set. The most competent or important dancers typically occupied the top place, whereas those who were
more hesitant or lesser in social significance generally stood at the sides
as the third and fourth couples. At the commencement of each figure, the
participants acknowledged each other in bows and curtseys while eight
bars of the tune were played. At less formal balls and later in the century,
this greeting was often dispensed with, although the musical introduction continued to function as a means of prompting kinetic memory and
acclimatizing dancers to a shift in rhythm and mood between each figure.
Earlier in the century, certain melodies were irrevocably associated with
specific figures, but in the last decade it became common to adapt popular tunes from the music hall, opera, or theatre. Each figure within the
Quadrille was composed of 8, 16, or occasionally 24 bars, lasting from two
to three minutes for all couples to complete. A whole set, including short
rests between each figure, took between 17 and 20 minutes to perform.

This choreographic structure allowed time for chatting, observation, and interaction with the other couples; it also enabled those less familiar with a particular figure to see it performed before embarking upon it themselves as their turn came around the set. The author of a ball room guide (Anon. [1874], p. 32) opined that 'though generally considered the slowest of dances, [it] is, perhaps, about the pleasantest and most sociable ever contrived'. The Quadrille's social character was much prized by those past the first flush of youth and who enjoyed conversation during the dance. Several authors commented upon how the Quadrille presented an opportunity to the elderly, the less physically able, and even the least competent of dancers to take part.

By the 1880s, however, the 'languid quadrille' was regarded by many as an 'intolerable bore', a response, arguably prompted by the loss of the Quadrille's more demanding steps in vogue during the early nineteenth century (Scott, 1887b, 1892; Crompton [1891]). Once embellished with steps drawn from the ballet repertoire, following the reforms of Parisian dancing master Cellarius in the 1840s, these more technical movements were replaced with a basic walking step, known as a *pas marché*. This step was performed with the foot a little turned out, a slight spring in the knee and instep, and a placing of the foot on the floor with the toe down first: such physical requirements tended to conserve energy while providing gentle exercise. Its frequent alternating appearance on typical ball room programmes afforded a welcome recuperative movement contrast to the dizziness of the Waltz.

Such a restrained dance, though, did not always suit the younger generation or those seeking more physical excitement in the ballroom. They preferred a much more energetic variant of the Quadrille, the Lancers, which took its name from the company of soldiers known as the Lancers who were famed for precise military drill manoeuvres. The Lancers Quadrille was first popular in the early 1820s, but enjoyed a revival from the middle of the century. Dancing teacher Mrs Henderson ([1879], p. 31) attributed its renewed attractiveness to the cultural lead of the state balls and 'corresponding circles in high life'. More important, no doubt, as a factor in its longevity was its quickly moving choreography and spirited music. Unlike the First Set, the figures of the Lancers 'do not afford such facilities for conversation, as the partners have frequently to separate, and there is not nearly so much time spent in waiting' (Scott, 1887a, p. 38). Although dancing teachers stressed the need to maintain straight lines, strict attention to musical phrasing, and clear execution of its swiftly moving evolutions, late-nineteenth century renditions of the

Lancers became the subject of heated exchanges (see Chapter 6) about declining standards of dancing and etiquette; the opportunity to exploit the choreography's potential for animated performances proved too tempting, especially for younger, physically fit dancers.

Within the category of square dances at large dance events, the Lancers had few rivals in popularity. The set of Quadrilles known as the Caledonians, for example, was considered more suitable for small-scale parties and tended to appear only once on an evening's ball, although it did maintain favour at Scottish balls.[2] To inject greater diversity into the repertoire and to improve their own business, dancing masters created fresh sets of Quadrilles that they hoped would capture the attention of fashionable society and endure for more than one season. Among the more successful were the *Polo Quadrille*, introduced into Britain from France, with additional figures by Robert Crompton; the *Prince Imperial's*, a particularly complicated set of figures that baffled even the experienced and enthusiastic dancer, Philip Richardson; and Edouard LeBlanc's composition, *La Nationale* [1883], which was appreciated, like the Lancers, for giving little respite to the dancers:

> [T]he sides are constantly employed in the dance, not standing still and watching the performance of the top couples till their turn comes, as in the old fashioned dance.[3]

La Nationale was distinctive in its use of English, Welsh, Scottish, and Irish melodies to accompany each of the four figures before concluding with that named the United Kingdom. The use of the Waltz step throughout *La Nationale* instead of the more usual *pas marché* met with success and, recognizing the late Victorians' fascination with waltzing, Crompton not only adopted this strategy in his own square dance composition, the Waltz Cotillon, but created its one and only figure to be performed throughout to waltz music.[4]

'The Queen of Dances': the Waltz

By the end of the nineteenth century, the Waltz was the single most important dance in the ball room. Gone were the negative responses it had encountered on its initial appearance in Britain, when there was widespread condemnation of the face-to-face position and the close physical embrace of the sexes. Fear of its supposed dangers of ill health, even possible madness, caused by the persistent whirling, had drawn extensive critical attention from parents, poets, and guardians of moral and public propriety. But its later favourable and frequent appearance in plays, novels, poetry, visual imagery, operettas, ballets, and music concerts testify to its acceptance as a valued dance form across most social classes in Europe, America, and colonial outposts.[5]

Above all, the Waltz was regarded as the ultimate dance of romance. As Scott (1887b, pp. 124–5), a respected analyst and commentator on the Waltz remarked from his perusal of contemporary fiction:

> I do not remember to have read a single pretty remark that was supposed to have been uttered while the couple were engaged in dancing a polka or schottische ... the hero, if he dances at all, is always a first-rate waltzer ... was there ever a heroine who did not waltz to perfection? And mark how the steps of the lovers are always in perfect unison.

Even in the late nineteenth century, however, the Waltz was not without its critics, not only on grounds of potential moral impropriety fostered by close bodily contact, but also on grounds of health. Criticism was voiced against the long hours of whirling in poorly ventilated and crowded rooms. Dedicated dancers with sufficient partners to choose from might theoretically cover 14 miles a night in waltzing around the room according to Scott (who advised wrapping up to keep warm in the night air when leaving and an early departure to benefit from a good night's sleep, 1887b, 1888). The general recommendation for waltzing was to regulate participation. Each Waltz set on the programme lasted for around 18 minutes at a time, but dancers chose to enter and leave the floor as they wished. This was essential not only to guard against tiredness, but also to prevent giddiness.

Over the years, numerous subtle variations in the performance of the Waltz appeared. To simplify, there were two principal versions in vogue at the end of the nineteenth century: the *Valse à Trois Temps* and the *Valse à Deux Temps*. Somewhat confusingly, 'temps' refers not to time but to the number of steps taken to each bar of three beats. In its earliest form in fashionable English society, the *Valse à Trois Temps*, as noted in the manuals of dancing master Thomas Wilson, used an evenly emphasized step pattern to the three beats of the bar. Later in the century, in response to the quickened pace and accent of the later Viennese-style waltz music, this was replaced by a greater emphasis on the first step of each bar. As Scott helpfully explains, the later preference was for a step matched by the syllables of 'wilderness'. Ever keen to provide 'modern' and 'scientific' analyses of dancing, Scott (1887b, p. 108) defined the 'Perfect Waltz' as

> a dance in triple time, of dactylic rhythm, consisting of six sliding steps, of which three are rotary, and three progressive and curvilineal – the curve described being of a cycloidal nature.

In spite of Scott's highly technical description of the 'Perfect Waltz' this was a comparatively simple choreographic structure to grasp or as happened in many instances to approximate rather than perfect. Performed with a slight turn-out of each leg from the hip, and pointed toes, the six movements took two bars of music, during which the couple effected one complete rotation on their axis while travelling forwards around the outer circumference of the room. Thus the dance consisted of one basic motif of three steps to a bar taking half a turn and was executed throughout using the ball room hold. This meant an unvarying spatial relationship and physical contact between partners that could also be used in other round dances. Ideally, the man drew his partner towards him as she stepped forwards, he backwards, initiating the propulsion. In the approved high-class style (see Figure 5.1), he supported the lady with his right hand above the left side of her waist, his left arm raised in a long curve to the side, his left hand gently holding her right hand. Depending on her height, the lady lightly rested her left hand on his right shoulder or upper arm, extending her right arm in a curve to join his left. Both dancers looked over the other's right shoulder and, in polite circles, maintained a respectful distance from each other's bodies.

A skilful partnership would exercise the 'graceful twinkling, playing in and out movement of the feet' (Scott, 1892, pp. 185–6) and, attentive to the physical laws of motion that Scott was at pains to analyse, attain the ideal of moving as one to relish the heady sensation of smooth, persistent circling. The Waltz came to symbolize a perfect union of heterosexual compatibility and union, popular opinion being encapsulated in the *London Illustrated Weekly* cartoon of 1889 which illustrates a variety of unsuitable partners from a female perspective (see Figure 5.2).

The *Valse à Deux Temps* enjoyed greater currency among the smart set surrounding the Prince of Wales from the 1880s and differed from the *Trois Temps* in that only two steps were taken (a step and close of the feet together most usually) occurring on the first and third beats of each bar. Especially useful in crowded ballrooms, the *Valse à Deux Temps* enabled dancers to change direction easily. A new pathway could be marked out by sideways steps, thus avoiding possible dizziness or collision with

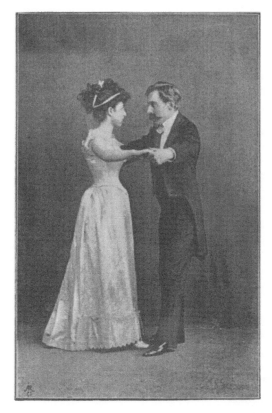

Figure 5.1   High Class Style, Edward Scott, *Dancing as an Art and Pastime*, 1892

other couples in the room. These problems would not have arisen if there was sufficient space in the ball room and, indeed, if every couple was competent enough to continue circling around the edges of the room equidistant from each other. 'Considering the long and immense popularity the waltz has enjoyed', observed Robert Crompton (1891, p. 49) 'it is surprising that really good waltzers are so very rare.' Such criticisms of contemporary waltzing are understandable from the pens of dancing masters, with more than a vested interest in condemning poor dancing. Yet the search for the perfect Waltz appears as a *leitmotif* in other instances of late Victorian discourse. For a dance that appeared so simple in its composition of one repetitive motif performed by just two people, the acquisition of the 'Perfect Waltz' was often viewed as the terpsichorean equivalent of the Holy Grail.

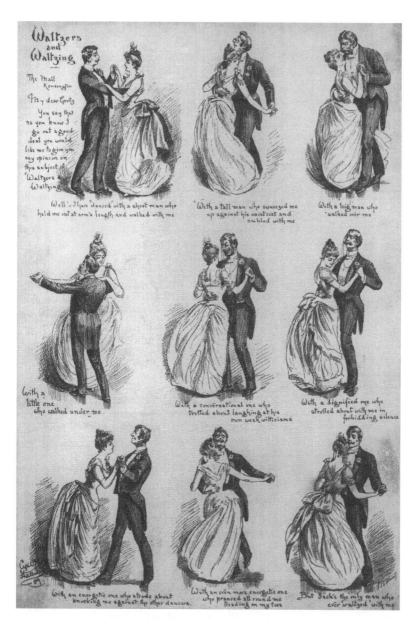

Figure 5.2 Waltzers and Waltzing, *Illustrated London News*, 1 January 1880

Diversity in the ball room

Poor waltzers had little escape in the late Victorian ballroom. Apart from sets of Quadrilles, there were few alternatives to what Scott dubbed the 'Queen of Dances' on the Society dance programme. At a royal ball in 1870 at Marlborough House, for example, of the 17 dances listed on the programme, the programme was evenly divided between Waltzes and Quadrilles, apart from a set of Lancers and a concluding Galop.[6] This pattern was typical of royal and Society balls over the next four decades, although at times, other couple dances such as the time-honoured Polka replaced the concluding Galop.

By the 1870s, the Polka, the rage of the 1840s, had settled into making occasional appearances on aristocratic programmes.[7] Like the Waltz, its earlier manifestations of various figures had been reduced to one rotary step motif in the ubiquitous ball room hold. Its 'really exhilarating and airy motion' (Crompton [1891], p. 13) remained to some extent in the distinctive 2/4 rhythm. Matching the musical pattern (Scott [1911, p. 132] likened it to saying 'a farm-yard here, a farm-yard there'), the Polka-step motif began with a hop or a rise on the upbeat of the preceding bar, followed by a transfer of weight on the first beat of the main bar. Two further steps were then taken on each note in the bar before recommencing the whole motif on the other foot. By the 1880s, the preliminary rise or hop was becoming lost and the dance rhythm flattened to three steps as dancers approximated the Waltz step to the Polka music. As a simple and rousing finale to a Society ball, another Parisian import from earlier in the nineteenth century was the Galop. Normally performed with a gliding step, followed by a chassé step, taken at speed to a fast, flowing 2/4 rhythm, the Galop had clear affinities in its foot patterns with the *Valse à Deux Temps*. The adoption of the *Valse à Deux Temps* was by no means obligatory for all dancers in court circles. The Princess of Wales herself was noted for her expert rendition of the *Valse à Trois Temps*.

By the Edwardian period, even the Polka and Galop had faded away, being replaced by the ubiquitous Waltz, just as they in turn had supplanted the old country dance *Sir Roger de Coverley*, once the inevitable closure to the ball, intended to bring young and old together on its longways formation. Lingering still at country balls, it was otherwise to be seen only at Christmas parties or at juvenile dances. In the 1870s, some country dances might be found scattered throughout the programme at metropolitan dances: notably *La Tempête*, which was organized in sets of four couples in longways formation, and *The Triumph*, a dance that had appeared since the late eighteenth century in numerous guises; its most distinctive figure of the lady flanked by a gentleman on either side, sometimes illustrated mid-century ball room guides.[8] In the concluding decades of the century, however, diversity in the ball room among the upper social level was best sought in the balls in Scotland or at the Caledonian Ball, which retained the Scottish preference for vigorous group dancing.[9] Indeed, it was a couple dance of supposed Scottish origin but undoubtedly from the continent, that remained in the repertoire. This was the *Schottische*, a couple dance performed in ballroom hold, in a distinctive 2/4 rhythm. It had variants such as the *Highland Schottische* in which the couple danced apart facing each other, raising an arm over the head, the other akimbo, in Highland style.[10] These forms had clear affinities with the succession of the later sequence dances invented by dancing masters and that became so popular among the lower-middle classes from the 1890s (see Chapter 7).

The first of the American imports, the *Barn Dance*, was clearly related in structure to the Schottische, as implied by its alternative names of the *Military Schottische* or *Schottische Militaire*.[11] It was by no means a new dance, nor did it have any association with barns, aside from the fact that in the United States, it was most often performed to a tune known as 'Dancing in the Barn'. In Britain, it found a place on many ball programmes, though notably it was not popular at court. Following acceptance in Society circles in 1888, it remained in currency throughout the social scale for about 20 years. One reason for its enthusiastic reception was its coupling with a well-known stage dance melody from the Gaiety Theatre, the *Pas de Quatre*, by which name it was often known, especially in Society circles. In the first part of its binary form, the couple stood side-by-side, either linking arms or holding hands, facing the line of dance around the room; in the second part, the dancers adopted the ballroom hold to turn and progress along the line of dance. The *Barn Dance*'s initial vogue owed much to the vigour and catchiness of its music, which was associated with popular performers, including the dancer Kate Vaughan at the fashionable Gaiety Theatre (D'Egville in Grove (1895)). Its spirit matched the desire for reinvigoration in the ball room especially among younger dancers; the choreography was easy to learn and any couple familiar with the Waltz and Quadrille could soon imitate other couples in the ball room.

Similar characteristics underlined the next craze from the United States: the *Washington Post* which was at the height of popularity in the winter season of 1895. Danced to a rousing march by American composer John Philip Sousa, the *Washington Post*, like its older cousin the *Barn Dance*, was structured in two parts. A distinctive feature of the dance was the couple's positioning in the first part. The woman stretched her left arm to the side, and raised her right arm slightly above her own right shoulder for the man to hold her left hand in his left, her right in his right, from his position behind and slightly to the left of her. According to Richardson (1960), the man then spent much of his time during the dance trying to avoid stepping on his partner's long dress.

More enduring in its popularity than the *Washington Post*, was the Two-Step, an American import that became widespread from the late 1890s and remained in fashion until the heyday of ragtime.[12] Initially, its accompanying music was not the syncopations of ragtime, but rousing marches by Sousa or similarly energetic music in 6/8 time. A comparatively easy dance, the Two-Step was closely allied to the earlier Galop. In the older dance, the chassé step had an uneven rhythm: the first sliding step of the chassé took longer to perform than the second closing step. In the Two-Step proper, both foot movements took equal time to perform. The appeal of the 6/8 rhythm, however, encouraged a variation in which dancers introduced three steps – the first two steps each taking half a beat and the third a full beat. Towards the end of the century, the first of the African-American sourced dances, the Cake Walk, had brief circulation among the middle classes (see Chapter 14).

Royal circles were resistant to any American introductions into their ballroom repertoire, preferring their staple diet of Quadrille, Waltz, Polka, and Galop, and the music of continental composers. From the 1880s, attempts were made to reinvigorate the repertoire not by embracing foreign forms from across the Atlantic but through quarrying historical dance forms of the old European courts. Attempts to introduce reconstructions of the Minuet, Gavotte, and Pavane met with a distinct lack of enthusiasm from regular social dancers. Amalgamations of detail from these older forms with elements of the Waltz, Quadrille, or other nineteenth-century dances were proffered by dancing masters: Scott's *Versa* (1892) for example, was inspired by the Minuet and Crompton's *Mignon* (1895) by the Mazurka. The latter's historically inspired *Minuet Valse* enjoyed some success in Britain, though it seems to have been particularly favoured on the continent.[14] These historically inspired dances also had a limited reception in Society, but the formula of composing new dances from existing familiar material proved exceptionally popular lower down the social scale. Standardization and comparative brevity were essential in social dance choreography for a clientele who had limited time and money at their disposal.

Collectively they came to be known as sequence dances, and in the twentieth and twenty-first centuries as 'old-time' or 'round dances'. These compositions fed the appetite of the keen lower-middle-class dancer for dances that could be easily learned yet were sufficiently new each season to pique the appetite. Typically constructed of 16 or 24 bars, they were usually constructed in two parts: the first part often on the spot, the second usually featuring a turning motif of the couple in typical progressive ballroom style. Classic examples are the *Veleta* and the *Military Two-Step*, each composed by dancing teachers who exhibited their compositions at the annual competitions for new dances run by dancing teacher societies during the late Victorian and Edwardian period. Such dances, as Richardson (1946) points out in his history of English ball room dancing, were perfect to cater for the hundreds of couples that frequented the assembly rooms and British seaside dance halls. The fixed choreography proved easy to memorize and the orderliness of composition meant that the limited space was used efficiently as all dancers followed on the same track. It was in the assemblies that the greatest variety of dances might be found in the late Victorian and Edwardian period, the repertoire narrowing higher up the social scale; it was also in this latter context that the greatest dissatisfaction was expressed at the standard of dancing.

6
Anarchy in the Ball Room

Merely a rowdy romp, men and youths dragging girls
about in the roughest manner, all looking hot and
blowsy. Is there no remedy?

An Old Fusilier, *The Morning Post*, 14 December,
1898, p. 3

Given the limited repertoire, the money and leisure to take lessons, and
the frequency of dance events, especially during the London Season, it
might be thought that the very best of social dancers in Britain at the
end of the nineteenth century might be found congregated in Society
circles. In fact, the opposite seems to have increasingly been the case.
There was even complaint about poor dancing standards at subscription
dances during the 1890s. Whereas in the past, dancers expected to learn
in childhood and annually renew their technique in order to participate
in the London Season, a one-off cheap course of dance lessons, usually
just in the Waltz, was often seen to suffice for many young men. Many
avoided full instruction in the whole repertoire, trusting to their limited tuition in waltzing, often acquired from a 'shilling hop' to enable
them to join in on the dance floor. In consequence, for those who went
to dances to fulfil social duties or purely to meet the opposite sex, the
niceties of choreographic distinction in the ball room repertoire were
meaningless, blurring all into one makeshift Waltz. Such levels of competence did not enthral those who took their dancing seriously.

Disorderly dancing

At numerous subscription events, experienced dancers objected to making up the Quadrille set with those they believed had received little or

no proper instruction. One complainant to *The Dancing Times* focused his wrath on the man in his set at an assembly dance who not only did not know the figures properly (he apparently 'slunk' and 'clutched' his way around) but insisted on waltzing through most of the dance. 'Waltzing at corners' in particular was disliked by traditionalists who objected to the 'interminable turn, twist, and whirl that goes on in our modern dancing.'[1] Hitherto, couples at the corners of the Quadrille set turned in a sedate manner by taking hold of both outstretched hands and performing the *pas marché* to circle on their own axis to the 4/4 or 6/8 music. This style of 'turning partners' remained in evidence at court balls and was favoured in aristocratic circles, especially among the older generation, for its decorum and its contrastive sensation to waltzing.

During the later century, however, the increasing pace of music, a characteristic of the German and military bands in vogue, drove dancers to rush to complete the turns at the corners of the set. Partially to remedy the undignified haste, partners began to turn in ball room hold, thereby cutting down on the amount of space required and consequently executing the turn more quickly. In a crowded ball room, such a strategy might be considered a sensible solution, but its adoption regardless of spatial conditions, often throughout the Quadrilles, brought forth vociferous complaints. Feelings with respect to the omnipresence of the Waltz in the ball room could run quite high. One dancer, signing himself 'Go As You Please', to the *Dancing Times's* correspondence columns in 1895 advocated a spirit of leniency, but an antagonist forcefully retorted

> I am a 16 stone muscular Christian, and warn "Go As You Please", that if he comes waltzing in my set and *I* go as *I* please, a hospital bed will be all he will want till the cricket season opens.[2]

Rowdyism

A far worse transgression in Society's eyes was the widespread dancing style christened by its opponents as 'romping' or 'rowdyism'. It first appeared as a target of frequent complaint in the 1880s when Society's younger generation were seen as the worst offenders; their unrefined behaviour was considered to be dangerously similar to that of the lower classes. Contemporary comments, however, suggest that young people in Society had little need of such models. For a generation less keen to attend regular dancing lessons, bored with the same dances on the programme, and possibly reacting physically and emotionally to the faster, spirited music then in fashion, the much-castigated romping style was

both fun and rebellious. The Countess of Ancaster, a high-profile aristocratic guardian of standards in social dancing, grumbled (in Grove,
1895, p. 416) that the

> young generation care for nothing but the wildest waltz or polka.
> There are at every ball good dancers, but, on the other hand, how
> many who cannot *dance* at all! They can hop and jump and make a
> great display of physical force, but this is not consistent with good
> taste, and is certainly not dancing.

Rowdyism was prevalent in the *Barn Dance*, the *Washington Post*, and
the Lancers. These dances were often vigorously performed by stamping
on the beat and lifting the legs higher than once considered decorous.
Toes were no longer elegantly pointed but raised in 'flat iron' position,
devoid of grace and in its force, consideration for other dancers. The
Lancers in particular lent itself to boisterous modes of execution. More
vigorous forms of this Quadrille were disparagingly referred to as the
Rowdy, Margate, or Kitchen Lancers, the titles of the two last suggesting the perceived provenance of the dance (Rogers, 2003). Edward Scott
(1892, p. 130) was in no doubt that London's stereotypical East End
working-class young man, 'Arry, was to blame for

> movements, for instance, as jigging around with both arms extended
> and hands clasped by the opposite dancer, turning backwards in the
> third figure of the Lancers, twisting partners round by the waist like
> so many whirligigs, and waltzing in the figures of set dances.

Regular complaints were voiced against the noise and vigour with
which the characteristic figure of *les lanciers* in this 'new war dance' as
Scott described it was performed:

> One thing, at least, may be said in favour of the final figure, which
> appears to be known by the very suggestive name of "Soldiers." It is
> distinctly characteristic. No sooner does it begin than the ball-room
> seems to be converted into a veritable pandemonium. A spirit of
> aggressive defiance pervades every movement. In place of the noise-
> less step of the dance proper, a pronounced and very audible martial
> tread is adopted throughout the figure, except only the action sug-
> gests a charge of cavalry. Adjacent sets are ruthlessly invaded, and
> no more regard is paid to the comfort and convenience of the ladies
> than might be expected in actual warfare.[3]

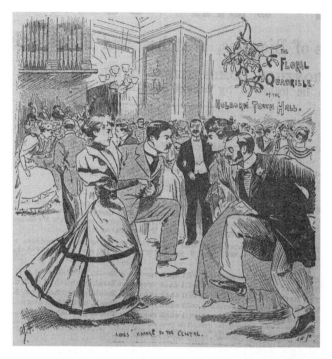

Figure 6.1   The Floral Quadrille, *The Penny Illustrated Paper*, 23 December 1893

A visual glimpse into how this figure was performed is given in the illustration of the Floral Quadrille as performed at Holborn Town Hall. The raised feet and hunched bodies are far from the erect figure and pointed toes advocated by dancing masters (see Figure 6.1).

Another site for anxiety lay in the exuberant renditions of the fourth figure of the Lancers where opposite couples meet in the centre of the set to circle round, the men placing their arms around the ladies' waists, and the ladies resting their hands on the shoulders of the man on either side. When performed at speed, it was not unusual for the women to lose their footing to end up 'swinging round like rag dolls'.[4] Not only did this cause discomfort to the ladies (though many undoubtedly enjoyed it), but other men standing in the set ran the risk of being kicked by the women: as one victim somewhat exaggeratedly described, 'in the middle of the back with both heels while rotating at the rate of forty miles an hour'.[5]

High-spirited renditions of the Lancers remained popular until well into the next century. Historian of dancing Reginald St Johnston in 1906

(p. 153) complained that 'a dozen people careering madly down the room, knocking aside all who may come in their way, at once destroys all the poetry of it'. At times it seems that the exuberance did get out of hand. There were reports of dancers being dragged by their hair and breaking limbs. As late as 1911, *The Lady* reported an incident in which one female dancer was dragged on the floor and kicked in the head.[6] Such physical damages were hardly a regular event, but their reportage helped to support the criticisms of poor and antisocial dancing which gained fresh impetus from responses to ragtime and later jazz.

Royalty certainly objected to the practice of romping and it never featured in the staid ceremony of state balls. Once a keen and able dancer Queen Victoria never appeared at public dances during the London Season following the death of Albert, though to the chagrin of the dancing profession south of the border, she did attend dances at Balmoral, if only to preside over them. Her son, the Prince of Wales, had enjoyed dancing in his younger days, and, if objecting to the practice of romping at Society events, he nonetheless was noted for spirited performances at his private gatherings. Indeed, one commentator went so far as to accuse Edward of validating an inferior style of technique so that the Waltz now 'resembled an old-fashioned rollicking gallop':

Is it possible that H.R.H., the Heir Apparent, is responsible for this change of pace during the past two years? *On dit* that the Prince can only dance the deux temps, and that, after an ineffectual attempt to revive the old-time scramble, he put on the pace of the present waltz to suit his regal trot.[7]

Pepping up the speed of the music was certainly a strategy in Society to provide 'go' in the fusty repertoire of Society dances, but in any case the fast-paced waltzes of the Strauss family and their ilk were favourites of Edward and Alexandra. George Grossmith, who had frequently observed Edward at play, also identified the Prince's waltzing as that of the 'deux temps' and described its performance within this circle as 'more or less of a gallop, at a gallop'.[8] Even less deferentially, further down the social ranks, dancing master and bandleader C. J. Melrose ([n.d.], p. 8) commented that, unlike George Grossmith, he himself had

not had the honour of hobnobbing with His Royal Highness, but if the description given by Mr. Grossmith be correct, truth compels me to express the treasonable opinion that H.R.H. is a poor sort of dancer. The site of the Prince's portly figure, "going it at a rate of thirteen to the dozen" must be a severe strain upon the loyal feelings of those faithful subjects who happen to be onlookers.

Around this time, the Prince had officially retired from full participation in dancing though his wife and certain members of his set continued.[9]
During the 1880s, the smart set embraced a revival of the Polka, dancing it with exuberance and vigour. Society entertainer George Grossmith, with a reputation as one of 'the most graceful of dancers' reported that the Polka

> is a great dance after supper in all the smartest circles. You should see them, as I have remarked *after* supper, going like mad, stamping and shouting and enjoying themselves to their hearts' content.[10]

Grossmith's lyrics to the infectious tune of his highly successful song, 'See Me Dance the Polka' (1887) underline the abandon and lack of decorum with which the dance was habitually performed:

> You should see me dance the Polka,
> You should see me cover the ground,
> You should see my coat-tails flying,
> As I jump my partner round;
> When the band commences playing,
> My feet begin to go,
> For a rollicking romping Polka
> Is the jolliest fun I know.

The pursuit of fun, though, was often at the expense of choreographic difference at the end of the century. Although the Polka's music and choreography were distinctive enough, the ubiquity of waltzing meant that the kinetic niceties of fitting specific foot motifs to the musical rhythm were frequently abandoned. Often the steps to the Polka lay beyond a young man's competence, the Waltz being his only ball room repertoire, as suggested in a *Punch* cartoon of 1885:

He.: It's a Polka; but we can waltz to it.
She.: Oh, not for worlds! I hate waltzing to a Polka: besides I adore the Polka step!
He.: Sorry, I –a-nevah dance the Polka; but we can sit out this dance, if you like – and *I will talk to you!*
She.: Oh, good gracious, no! Let us dance it *anyway you like!*[11]

In any case, the Polka was thought not conducive to romance, being considered 'too hoppy and skippy' for sweet nothings to be murmured into the fair partner's ear.[12] Regardless of its inappropriateness for courtship, the Polka's revival highlights growing frustration with the monotony of waltzing and a widespread desire to find a more exhilarating dance to enliven the familiar proceedings.

The issue of reversing

It was not, however, only sheer boredom at the number of Waltzes on a Society programme that caused dissatisfaction among Society, but a more physically disorientating feature of the dance proved to be a problem. One of the most contested aspects about waltzing correctly was the issue of 'reversing'. Most commonly, on commencing to waltz, couples revolved clockwise on their own axis progressing anti-clockwise around the ball room; reversing meant, quite simply, changing the direction of turn to anti-clockwise, as the couple continued to move forwards along the line of dance. It was a useful technique to provide variety in the dance.[13] More crucially, it prevented the dancers from becoming dizzy, without having recourse to leaving the dance floor to steady themselves after incessant whirling in one direction.

The concept, however, was easier than the reality of its execution. To be effective at reversing required knowledge, competence, and confidence on the part of the man to steer his partner appropriately, but it also needed skill and understanding from the woman in knowing how to respond to her partner's bodily signals. It was a technique, Scott insisted and no doubt rightly, that required proper instruction and practice outside of the ball room to prevent potential collisions. To be effective, the man needed to maintain a tight embrace of his partner while indicating to her through the placement of his left foot between her feet, pressure on her waist via his left arm and hand, and a strong steer to the left, that he was reversing the direction of the turn. Given these indicators, a good female dancer could follow but all too often, hesitant men were doomed to failure when they approached the shift in direction verbally.

More than presenting physical difficulties to late-nineteenth-century dancers, the art of reversing also carried social significance. In Society circles, it was popularly considered 'bad form' to reverse. There are a complex of reasons for this: firstly, as Scott (1892) suggests, the necessity of holding the woman very close, in order to effect the turn, might have been found objectionable in certain circles; secondly, few men bothered to learn how to reverse, and displays of competence in the manoeuvre called unwanted attention to the brave man who, unlike his Society fellows, had spent time at the dancing class; and thirdly, reversing in front of royalty at state balls was just not allowed. This last factor may have been consequent upon the first and second: court society no doubt preserved aristocratic codes of proximity on the most formal of occasions and, if the standard of dancing among aristocratic men in general was so poor, the ban may have arisen to prevent the embarrassment of likely collisions in the royal presence.[14]

American high society had no such qualms, their dancers being renowned for ease of execution in the technique of reversing and, indeed, for their general dancing accomplishment. The disparity in technical ability between the home-grown dancers and the visitors was undoubtedly a cause of frustration to the latter. Canadian novelist and journalist Sara Jeanette Duncan (1891, pp. 177–8) offers both a female and New World perspective in her gently satirical portrait of English Society dancing:

> We inserted ourselves into the moving mass, and I went hopelessly round the Maypole that Mr Mafferton seemed to have turned into, several times. Then the room began to reel. "Don't you think that we had better reverse?" I asked, 'I am getting rather dizzy, I'm afraid.' Mr Mafferton stopped instantly, and the room came right again. 'Reverse?' he said, 'I don't think I ever heard of it. I thought we were getting on capitally.' And when I explained to him that reversing meant turning round, and going the other way, he declared that it was quite impracticable – that we would knock everyone else over, and that he had never seen it done. After the last argument I did not press the matter. It took very little acquaintance with Mr Mafferton to know that if he had never seen it done, he never would do it.

In this publication lie clues to the fourth reason for the absence of reversing from Society: reversing was a characteristic move among the London upper-middle class, not Society. Their style was mocked by Grossmith both in his 1889 interview for the *Pall Mall Gazette* and also more directly in his comic song 'See Me Reverse' ([1884]).[15] It is difficult to appreciate the humour of this song today without some knowledge of both the social context and the kinetic niceties of contemporary waltzing. Grossmith's credentials for commenting on the various dance styles of the day were cited by his interviewer: 'you are one of the crack dancers in town; you go everywhere, you see everything, you dance a hundred steps.' This interview, together with the lyrics of his song, records stylistic movement details of the waltzing of a social group who were to contribute to lasting changes in ball room technique, even if during the 1880s such ways of moving appeared risible to those in the upper echelons of fashion. The Pooterish character of Grossmith's 'dancing man' in 'See Me Reverse' derives its humorous appeal from the seriousness and snobbery with which he pursues his enthusiasm for dancing, his competence in which is based on a meagre course of cheap lessons taken the year before. This reverser was quite clearly a type recognizable to fashionable audiences of the time:

> I think I may venture to say,
> You all must have seen me by chance,
> I'm monarch of all I survey
> At ev'ry subscriptional dance.
> I waltz with an amiable smile,
> My remarks are most simple and terse
> I slither in stiff poker style,
> With a swagger attempt to reverse.
> Chorus
> *And the hearts of all damsels I storm*
> *With my Nor'west South Kensington Form.*
> *So watch me gently gliding*
> *O'er the parquet sliding;*
> *And now and then colliding,*
> *And see me reverse.*

The reverser is a fashionable young man or 'masher' whose families typically resided in the enclaves of Kensington, Bayswater, and Notting Hill. Positioned socially and geographically on the edges of Society, the families of the Kensington Gores, Bayswater Browns, and Notting Hill Joneses, as Grossmith caricatures them, had adopted a distinctive waltz style, introduced by their young men. The languid musical accompaniment of 'See Me Reverse' apes the 'funeral' pace beloved of this contingent of waltzers who, according to Grossmith, 'thinks it *bad* form to let itself go, and never relaxes its rigidity and its frigidity for a moment'.[16] A further trait of the dancing of the upper-middle class, according to Grossmith, was their repudiation of the older 'off the toe' style of dancing favoured by Society. In contrast, the upper-middle class preferred to slide their feet in an exaggerated manner on the flat foot without turning the toes outwards. This habit of gliding 'as melancholy as mutes at a funeral' Grossmith observed, was purely an affectation peculiar to their class. He did pay these dancers the compliment of being good at steering their partners around the room, but condemned what he regarded as their semaphore or poker style of ball room hold, in which the dancers' outstretched arms were held out stiffly at a right angle to the body. Teachers, he was convinced, merely enforced local custom, though his belief that the style ultimately derived from Boston is worthy of further reflection with respect to the development of the dance of that name during the early 1900s (see Chapter 13).

In practice, even within Society drawing rooms, there were many variations of the Waltz, some of which made appearances under distinctive names, taken either from their manner of execution, such as the Hop Waltz or Spring Waltz, or, more satirically, from their supposed provenance, as in the Liverpool Lurch, the Ratcliffe Highway Kick, and the Kensington Crawl. Caricatured by *Punch* (see Figure 6.2) and condemned by Scott (1887a), these deviations from the preferred Society style were marked as either low class or provincial.

Civilization on the wane

In 1902, the London correspondent of the *Glasgow Herald* reported that

> the decline in dancing has only been in the great world of Society, not among the upper classes who are well-to-do without being in Society, not among the middle classes, not among the working classes.[17]

This opinion was shared by many. By the 1890s, there was a real sense that the Upper Ten were failing in their duty to act as models of civilized behaviour. Society hostesses complained that dancers lower down the social scale surpassed their superiors in technique and decorum. 'The middle classes put us to shame' lamented one correspondent to the *Morning Post*, noting their willingness, unlike Society, to take regular dance classes. Even in the East End of London, home to the poor, to workers and to immigrants, 'the "masses" entirely eclipsed the "classes" in the art of dancing'.[18] This verdict was delivered by 'A Primrose Dame', an aristocratic member of the Primrose League, the late-nineteenth-century society founded to uphold and spread the principles of the Conservative party. In her experience, East Enders considered that 'express speed, consequent collisions and rowdiness were ... vulgar', whereas in smart Society ball rooms such measures had become the norm. This *volte face* was also evident in the countryside: '[o]ne's own gardeners and village-lads seem completely puzzled at the "upper's" excessively bad dancing'.[19]

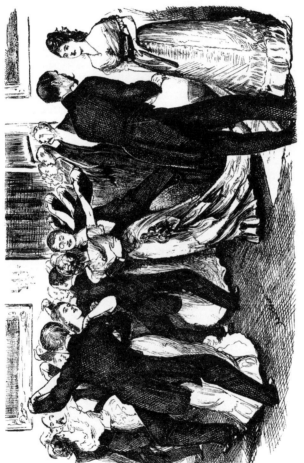

WHAT OUR WALTZING IS COMING TO.

Distinguished Foreigner. "VOULEZ-VOUS ME FAIRE L'HONNEUR DE DANSER CETTE VALSE AVEC MOI, MESS MATILDE?"

Miss Matilda (an accomplished Waltzer). "AVEC PLAISIER, MONSIEUR. QUELLE EST VOTRE FORME—LE 'LURCH DE LIVERPOOL, LE 'DIP DE BOSTON', OU LE 'KICK DE RATCLIFFE HIGHWAY?'"

[*We have feebly tried to represent the "Ratcliffe Highway Kick," which at present is only danced in the very best society, and confers a great air of distinction on the performers.*]

Figure 6.2   What Our Waltzing Is Coming To, *Punch*, 29 January 1876

At the village dances, a diverse repertoire prevailed, whereas members of the smart set, if they danced at all, favoured the more simplistic *Barn Dance, Washington Post* and riotous renditions of the Lancers. Higher up the social scale, it was only in the smart functions of the upper-middle classes, in establishments like the Carlton Restaurant, that a 'perfect dance' might be witnessed where 'people do really dance' (Machray, 1902, p. 93). Indeed, more diligent application to dance technique might be witnessed at the lower-middle-class shilling hops at Holborn Town Hall. Perhaps, as Machray acutely observed, the lack of enthusiasm here for the Cake Walk with its simplistic steps and invitation to dance with 'abandon' ran counter to the self-image and aspirations of a class of people who were intent on improving their social standing (see Chapter 14).

It had been hoped in some quarters that the increasing influx of the *nouveaux riches* into Society with their 'vigorous sons and daughters' might act as a spur to reverse the decline in Society dancing. Newly rich parents ensured that their offspring were fully schooled in dancing and deportment, but 'patrician society, the old families, often with pedigrees longer than their purses, would not take dancing lessons from mere millionaires'.[20] British Society expected to lead not to follow. The Primrose Dame's suggestion that Society might adopt more socialist leanings in following the example of the lower classes went unheeded, for the time-honoured practice of imitation of aristocratic lifestyles by the 'merely wealthy and the middle classes' was unlikely to be reversed, particularly at a time when the 'idle rich' felt increasingly threatened politically and economically by those below their station.

By the end of the century, the Society ball room, once held as the epitome of decorum and civilized recreation, was compared with a nursery or playground. The dancers, according to Scott,[21] had progressed little beyond children's games such as 'Here we go round the Mulberry Bush' (in the Lancers) and playing at horses (*Washington Post*). Here too, Scott argued, was worrying evidence of Max Nordau's theory of degeneration in the arts. Dancing, once the pursuit of men of consequence, was now the pastime of women and children; the art was declining towards an ever greater simplicity, a state of affairs that worryingly suggested the symptoms of decline in a once great civilization.

The *leitmotif* of degeneration echoed across most aspects of late Victorian life as the end of the century neared. Britain's political and economic supremacy in the world and that of its aristocratic leaders came under increasing threat in the century's closing decades. From beyond its shores, challenges to imperial acquisitions and ambitions came from France, Germany, and the Boers, while within the country, quickening social mobility and rapid population growth among the urban work force nurtured millenialist fears for the stability of the old order. Alongside letters of complaint in the London press about declining standards in the ball room might be found cries of alarm expressed by the social elite about the difficulties of finding servants and the decline of good manners.

Antidotes to anarchy

Nostalgia for the past was endemic in Victorian life, particularly in the arts. The Victorians turned to the seeming security of the past as a resource for their spiritual, aesthetic, and social present, almost as an antidote to the rapid advances being made in science and technology that were transforming the landscape and social relations (Lowenthal, 1985; Readman, 2005). Such cultural primitivism, viewing the past as superior to the present day, was discernible in the many reflections on contemporary dancing. The dancing of earlier generations, correspondents to the *Daily Graphic* in 1891 bemoaned, was so much more energetic and intergenerational. The illustrator Phil May captured this communal idyll of Regency times in 'How our Grandfathers Danced', a cartoon in which men and women, both young and old, dance a Quadrille in a sprightly and co-operative manner. The contrastive image May positioned below is labelled 'How we do not dance' and depicts the ball room of his own era where the sexes sit or stand around the edges of the ball room, alone, talking, or looking bored.[22]

May's choice of the early 1800s period to serve as a point of comparison with the present was by no means random. Not only did it chime with continuing Victorian enthusiasm for the world of Thackeray's *Vanity Fayre* (1848), but it also recalled the more central role that dancing played in aristocratic relations. May was not alone in turning to the Regency, a period for late Victorians that lay on the fringe of living memory. The Regency ball room, liberally interpreted, was a frequent subject for a European genre of late Victorian art that looked back more generally to the eighteenth century. It was popularized in Britain by painters such as Royal Academician Sir William Quiller Orchardson whose 1884 painting 'Her First Dance' (now in the Tate Collection) represents an imagined ball room scene of around 1820.

Beyond the strict dates of the Regency, the imagery of the eighteenth century proved a source of inspiration across a variety of late Victorian and Edwardian cultural forms. Aristocratic and well-to-do ladies and gentlemen in powder, wigs, and panniers stare out from the late Victorian Society press, in a portrayal perhaps of their own ancestors, recorded at a costume or historical ball, fixed by the studio photographer or illustrator. Sometimes that ancestry might have been more imagined than real, as in the case of upper-bourgeois married couple Maud and Leonard Messel. Dressed as eighteenth-century singer and hypothetical forebear Elizabeth Linley and dramatist Richard Brinsley Sheridan, they attended the Chelsea Arts Ball in 1911, wearing actual eighteenth-century costume from Maud's historical costume collection. Among their artist friends, they counted eighteenth-century genre painter Marcus Stone and historical-genre painter and collector of historical costume Talbot Hughes, as well as Percy McQuoid, illustrator of Lilly Grove's *Dancing*.[23] As art historians Hook and Poltimore (1986, p. 295) have argued, the eighteenth century 'assumed an almost mythic significance for bourgeois Europe of a hundred years later', as the newly rich looked back to an ostensibly more civilized and leisured world. Powdered and bewigged young lovers and dancers in eighteenth-century costume recur in late Victorian and Edwardian illustrations and on the professional and amateur stage, examples of the wider artistic vogue known as the Queen Anne Movement which, more broadly than its name suggests, involved an eclectic mix of historical elements (Girouard, 1977).

That imaginative mix and sense of revivalism extended to dancing. In the 1880s, recreations of seventeenth- and eighteenth-century balls in France included revivals of the Minuet and Gavotte (Vuillier, 1898), a fashion soon followed by English Society hostesses at their balls. Robert Crompton's Renaissance Dance Troupe gave exhibitions at numerous private and subscription balls in London, his high profile in such work leading to his nickname of Robert 'Minuet' Crompton. The golden age of the dancing master looked set to return as the demand for Minuets and Gavottes was followed by demand for dances of an earlier age, the Pavanes of the Elizabethan period and the mediaeval Branle. The national craze for historical pageantry and the late Victorian and Edwardian Shakespearean revival (Buckley, 1911) prompted further impetus to the fashion for historical dances (Holt, 1907).

One of the most high profile supporters of the movement was Mrs Cornwallis West (Lady Randolph Churchill) who played the piano for performances of the early music and dance revivalist Nellie Chaplin and her sisters, who along with Mabel Dolmetsch, wife of early music pioneer Arnold Dolmetsch, prompted more rigorous scrutiny of historical sources for dance.[24] Earlier, theatrical choreographers John D'Auban and Robert Crompton drew upon texts in the British Library for their versions of Minuets. Scott, however, as a more assiduous dance historian, was scathing about the frequent bowing and curtseying of these theatricalized forms; in his judgement, they revealed insufficient demonstration of sustained balance and grace and ignorance of primary sources. Authenticity, however, in spite of the rhetoric and intention of leading champions of the historical dance revival was not the principal concern of most Society dancers who were content to view reconstructions through the sentimental gauze of the Queen Anne Movement.[25]

Hope was expressed that these dances of a more civilized and elegant past might both rekindle interest in social dancing and provide models of decorum for the young to emulate. But as Louis D'Egville observed of Pavanes, Minuets, and Gavottes (in Grove, 1895), the lack of standardization in teaching them and the excessive length (in the case of the Menuet de la Cour) in effect rendered these dances useless in the ball room.

Robert Crompton continued to hold out hope for historical dances, taking inspiration from the German court where Kaiser Wilhelm II had approved the inclusion of Minuets and Gavottes at the court balls. In 1909, only two waltzes appeared on the programme at the German court, unlike in Britain where they dominated every court dance event. Crompton, in his role as President of the Imperial Society of Dance Teachers, together with Charles D'Albert, the Secretary, wrote to King Edward to request that 'at least, one State Ball during the coming Season, [be] arranged to include a revival of the elegant Court Dances of former periods.'[26] Beyond a bland acknowledgement of receipt, however, the letter secured no change.[27] It was in any case doubtful by now that the Edwardian court could wield any change in the fashionable ball room. Historical dances became more of a cult genre and the attempts to promote English country dances by revivalists Nellie Chaplin, Alice Cowper Coles, and Cecil Sharp similarly fell on stony ground in the ball room. The young of the ruling classes did not want to be civilized; they wanted to have fun, and that fun might well be found far away from the ball room of their parents and grandparents.

Part II
Fashioning Gentility

7
A Noble Profession

to refine and cultivate the taste of pupils, to ennoble our
profession and gain the respect of our fellow creatures.
Edward Scott, *Dancing as an Art and Pastime*,
1892, p. 214

Learning how to dance and how to behave at a late Victorian Society ball
required the services of an expert dancing teacher. Since the days of the
Italian Renaissance, dancing masters had been employed by European
royalty and aristocracy to fashion a socially distinctive body, trained
from childhood in regal deportment and in the court dances of the day.
The political and social significance of this 'artful body' as French cultural historian Sarah R. Cohen (2000) has termed it, reached its zenith at
the seventeenth-century court of Louis XIV. Its powerful traces continued to resonate over the succeeding centuries, as a visible symbol of what
it meant to embody the lifestyle and values of the social elite. In the
long-lasting wake of cultural influence that flowed across Europe from
Versailles, French taste and manners in bodily display led the fashionable
world until late in the nineteenth century.[1]

Paris remained the epicentre for the latest in dancing styles; its salons
and theatres acting as a crucible in which new ideas were refined according to aristocratic taste; these were then disseminated across what were
held to be the civilized countries of Europe, America, and their empires.
In Britain, as elsewhere in this cultural circuit, a dancing master or mistress who was annually able to refresh their knowledge directly from the
Parisian source commanded greater respect and income than those provincial, or less resourceful, dancing teachers whose contact with fashion
was often several times removed. Advertising a recent return from Paris
was a regular strategy to attract the gentry and bourgeoisie. The latest

dances and styles of performing the repertoire were cascaded down the pedagogic chain from a few influential individuals or families whose French connections were well established and constantly replenished. Other dancing teachers of repute among Society were famous professional dancers, either retired or between theatrical contracts, possessing careers in the first tier of European opera houses, whether Milan, Rome, Vienna, London, or Paris. Given the cultural pre-eminence of the court and the London Season, the most respected and prosperous of dance pedagogues could be found residing in the capital's West End.

Unsurprisingly in this class-obsessed society, teachers of dancing and deportment were ranked in a pyramidal structure that was closely tied to the social strata for whom they worked: like many service industries in the period, the profession of dance pedagogy reflected the tastes, fashions, and hierarchical social structure of its pupils. At the apex of the profession stood the privileged few, who taught a regular clientele of royalty and the grand aristocracy. Below these were the well-to-do teachers who operated from premises in central London to cater principally to the upper-middle classes. Then, in descending scale of influence came the many London teachers who taught classes and organized dances for the lower-middle class. At the bottom of the scale lay a whole range of dance teachers whose tuition and repertoire possessed little prestige, varied in quality, and was often a means of supplying a secondary income.

The majority of urban teachers followed the long-established practice of regular teaching from autumn through to early summer, holding weekly classes at their own premises and travelling to schools and private homes in the vicinity. Beyond this, in a long-established practice, summer months in the dancing teacher's year were devoted to knowledge and skills refreshment, at home or abroad, the more successful teachers occasionally tutoring provincial or less informed colleagues.[2]

Typically, the dancing teacher of late Victorian England was proficient across four areas: he or she taught dances from the current ball or drawing room repertoire; 'fancy dances', a term meaning the various short solos, duets, trios, or small group dances mostly adapted from the stage for amateurs to perform; instruction in deportment so that individuals could move elegantly in social life; and more general physical exercises, often grouped under the heading of callisthenics, which were designed to promote good health and a graceful figure. In the rural provinces, the teacher's repertoire was virtually identical with that taught in London, although it might well include some of the older country dances, or in Scotland the reels and strathspeys that were popular during the winter season.[3] Aristocratic families returning to the capital each year usually visited a London Society teacher early in the Season to remain abreast of the fashion, or they sometimes attended special rehearsals to learn the figures for a ceremonial Quadrille at a special ball.[4]

For royalty, aristocracy and the more London-orientated gentry, such lessons were a renewal and expansion of their existing competence in dancing and a style of deportment that had been acquired from an early age. Following the practices of the eighteenth-century social elite, the dancing teacher was responsible for socializing individuals into the repertoire and conduct expected at a court ball or Society dance, and for nurturing the healthy physical development of their young pupils. Although some adults did learn fancy dances and participate in physical exercises later in the nineteenth century, these aspects of a dancing teacher's trade were deemed more suitable for young, growing bodies, and as an important aid to the incorporation of social values.

The children of British royalty and aristocracy were systematically taught at home in their country stately houses, as well as in their London mansions where they often formed classes made up of their peers, or else attended the select classes of a Society teacher. At the children's parties and afternoon Society 'at homes', the younger boys and girls might perform a selection of fancy dances. Some of these dances had long histories, their choreographies passed across generations of teachers. As well as providing enjoyment, they were important means of embodying notions of gender, class, and national identities among the young (see Chapters 10 and 12). Evergreen examples from the fancy dance repertoire were the Sailor's Hornpipe, Highland Fling, Irish Jig, Fan Dance, and Tambourine Dance. During the late 1880s and 1890s, the Skirt Dance, Step dancing, and various dances revived from the past such as the Minuet, Pavane, and Gavotte were in vogue especially among young women (see Chapter 12).

Young people not only performed fancy dances for enjoyment and display but also as physical exercise to promote good health. The Victorians were obsessed with the pursuit of health, even those accustomed to better standards of nourishment and life conditions (Haley, 1978). Regardless of class, high infant mortality, frequent deaths of mothers in childbirth, deadly epidemics, poor air quality in the cities, and a high incidence of tuberculosis and other wasting diseases were widespread challenges. Consequently, it is not surprising that the wealthier Victorians paid considerable attention to various modes of physical training to achieve the growth of healthy lungs in a strong and upright body.

Wealth and social station introduced aristocratic and upper-class children to forms of physical self-expression far removed from those meted out to their counterparts in the lower echelons of society. When and where physical training was incorporated into schooling among the poor, it most often took the form of drill, the playground being employed as a site for formation marching rather than dancing to music.[5] Rich children, in addition to learning drawing room and fancy dances, were taught exercises to promote health and graceful ease of movement. As Sheila Fletcher, historian of women's physical education in Britain has pointed out (1984), the Greek etymology of callisthenics, means 'beautiful strength', attributes considered particularly desirable for well-bred women, rather than for the working population whose aesthetic considerations were often deemed irrelevant by their social superiors.

The dancing teacher had long made claims for the beneficial effects of dancing on the physique,[6] and callisthenics, rather than gymnastics or drill, formed part of their tuition. Variable in content according to the teacher's taste, knowledge, and clientele's interests, callisthenics embraced exercises performed mostly on the spot, such as knee bends, rises on the toes, low leg lifts, lifting and circling the arms, bending the body from the waist, and marching in group formations. Specialist equipment might also be deployed: lifting and lowering light-weight dumb bells while standing, and the use of a chest expander device designed to promote healthy lungs and, for girls, a firmer bustline.[7] Whatever the particular system, callisthenics as practised by English dancing teachers appears to have been predominantly non-aerobic: the idea of working up a sweat was antithetical to Victorian notions of ladylike conduct and was thought injurious to the health of the very young and the female. Dismissive of violent exercise in their championing of grace and beauty, many dancing teachers were equally opposed to the use of apparatus designed to improve the range of movement or increase exertion. Nonetheless a number of prominent Society teachers did employ Indian clubs or skipping ropes in their classes. Leonora Geary's advertisements often referred to her 'celebrated Indian Sceptre exercises' and Society teacher Mrs Wordsworth was later credited with the introduction of skipping ropes into her dance classes, possibly influenced by the popularity of skipping-rope dances at the Gaiety Theatre in the 1870s.[8]

Moving as ladies and gentlemen

An erect posture and easy mobility not only indicated the state of health of a person but also his or her social class: a better-fed and rested aristocracy, unbowed by the physically harsh work demands of earning a living, whether in the fields or factories, was generally taller and heavier than their social inferiors. This upright gait and air of confidence were further inscribed into the body by the dancing teacher's lessons in deportment. During the nineteenth century, cultural ideals of gentlemanly and ladylike movement and posture had become less mannered in British polite society. English taste in deportment had moved further and further away from the stylized movement of the French court. Instead, aristocratic ladies and gentlemen avoided what was perceived as the studied and ostentatious manners of the French in favour of a restrained and quiet style of social interaction that was considered natural and that did not draw attention to the performer.

More formalized ways of moving were considered to be artificial and disingenuous, ill-suited to the character of a modern, entrepreneurial nation that now outranked France. Contemporary appraisal of this redundant style of studied deportment is captured in responses to Dickens's character of Turveydrop, the dancing master in *Bleak House* (1853) who, although admired for his bodily command of the older style of deportment, personifies useless and insincere anachronisms. Correct ways of moving and standing still counted in social circles, however, even if the Turveydrop school of deportment was dismissed by late Victorian commentators on dancing and deportment as old-fashioned and risible.[9] Where the teaching of deportment lingered longest was for the conservative rituals of the court, in particular that of court presentation, for which Society teachers offered special classes (see Chapter 9). More typically, lessons primarily amounted to

> how to walk without looking like a tired camel, or an apprehensive penguin ... how to bow without giving the impression of a hen pecking at a worm; how to shake a hand without wringing it, or holding it aloft as though airing it, or at a distance as though it smelt, and how to enter a room with ease and dignity ... In other words, how to look like ladies and gentlemen.
>
> (D'Egville, 1937, p. 1)

Society dance teachers

Among the most sought-after dancing teachers in late Victorian England were former ballerina Marie Taglioni, dancing master Louis D'Egville and his son Louis, and teacher of dance and physical culture, Mrs Wordsworth. The large clientele of the latter was drawn principally from the young family members of the more socially mixed and expanded Society as well as those of the aristocratic order. The D'Egvilles, father and son, and Taglioni principally restricted their social dance tuition to royalty and the greater aristocracy.

Taglioni (1804–84) in her prime had been the favourite dancer of Queen Victoria and following retirement from the stage in 1848, continued to be hailed as a living legend. From 1872 to 1880, she periodically rented a house close to the prestigious locality of Mayfair, where she gave classes and private lessons to the children and adults of the British court. To ensure exclusivity, the names of commoners attending the classes at which royals were present were always passed to the Queen for prior approval. The most important source on Taglioni's London teaching is the diary of child pupil Margaret Rolfe, whose writings, sketches, and paintings provide unique insight into the latter years of this famous ballerina. Rolfe's diary and later reminiscences depict the working life of a well-positioned late Victorian dancing mistress in London and provide a rare glimpse into the lessons in dance and deportment of British royalty. Rolfe also shares her reflections on relations between royalty and commoners, between young and old, on amateur and professional dancers, and on the conventional restrictions placed upon young women. Such personal observations from pupils are all too rare, the portrait owing much to the singular relationship between Rolfe and Taglioni, enhanced by family friendship, the pupil's love and talent for dance, and Taglioni's fame and reputation as a figure worthy of recall and documentation for posterity.[10]

Apart from Taglioni's comparatively brief appearances as a teacher in London, the most prestigious of royal teachers, were those from the D'Egville Michau dynasty of whom Louis D'Egville the elder (1819–92) and younger (1852–27) enjoyed particular fame. Cited in various upper-class biographies and memoirs, the D'Egvilles belonged to a dancing family that traced a professional lineage stretching back to the court of Louis XIV.[11] Few teachers could compete with such credentials. Not without bias, members of the family asserted that they were

> the only ones who knew anything about the art, the only ones who, by right of heredity, had earned the monopoly. They had done it for generations.
>
> (D'Egville, 1937, pp. 5–6)

Louis the elder benefited from the knowledge and connections of his aunt, the 'celebrated Mme Michau'. Born Sophia D'Egville, Mme Michau (c. 1783–1859) was the sister of the famous James D'Egville, friend of Byron, professional dancer, esteemed choreographer, and founder of the first, if short-lived ballet school in London. Mme Michau played a vital role as *maîtresse de ceremonies* for the Prince Regent's court balls and dances in the early nineteenth century, and was later widely acknowledged as the undisputed expert on royal and aristocratic deportment. Moving between family houses in London and Brighton, following the seasons of fashionable Society, by the 1840s Mme Michau and her family had built a reputation and clientele that was admired and envied by many within the pedagogic profession.[12] As her most successful professional heir, Louis the elder had no need to re-locate each season to find pupils. To their house 'every great family in the country sent its women and most of its men' (D'Egville, 1937, p. 4). When Louis D'Egville, father and son, left their home to teach it was usually to visit the likes of Buckingham Palace and Montagu House (Stewart, 1938), not the village halls, public houses, and school rooms that so many less-fortunate peripatetic teachers frequented (see Figure 7.1).

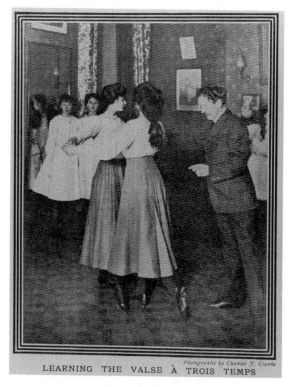

LEARNING THE VALSE À TROIS TEMPS

Figure 7.1 Learning the *Valse à Trois Temps* (Louis D'Egville) *The Tatler*, 18 January 1911

Although in effect servants to the court, both D'Egvilles spent leisure time with high-ranking aristocracy. As founder and leader of an amateur largely aristocratic orchestra, Louis the elder played alongside Lord Gerald Fitzgerald, Lord Chelmsford, and the Earl of Wilton. Both father and son were gifted violinists and composers, the son also later writing music for the theatre.[13] His family's artistic life was rich, counting professional dancers and visual artists among visitors to their home, as well as attracting musical celebrities such as Artur Rubenstein, and relatives of Charles Dickens and Joseph Strauss.

The third most renowned London teacher during this period, Mrs Wordsworth (1843–1932) did not boast such easy social connections with royalty and aristocracy, even if she reportedly took care to court the attention of the titled mothers who were allowed to observe the progress of their children during her classes (De Valois, 1957). *The Dancing Times* in 1911 noted that there could be

> few of the leaders of society during the past half century who have not at some time or other come under her tuition.[14]

She commuted daily to her school in South Kensington, enjoying a rural retreat in a large house with her retired London solicitor husband, four children, and five servants. The daughter of a well-to-do family of dancing teachers from Brighton, she exercised a commanding presence and was quick to spot errors in spite of potential limitations of a diminutive stature and visual impairment. Like many Society and upper middle-class daughters, Ninette de Valois (1898–2001) ballerina, choreographer, and founder of England's Royal Ballet, began her early dance career under the tutelage of Mrs Wordsworth. In her autobiography (1957, p. 28) she paints a vivid picture of Mrs Wordsworth entering a dance class:

> [I]n sweeps a plump, dumpy old lady. What an entrance! – the long black silk dress ending in a train, lace at the throat, tiny plump hands encased in short white kid gloves crossed over the stomach, and a lace handkerchief dangles from two fingers. The figure is erect, imposing, possibly modelled on Queen Victoria; it resembles a neat little yacht in full sail. 'Dance it, children … dance it' – the voice is a siren rising above the music. Rows of small heads are held higher and skirts are played with greater zeal, and the gathering of mothers would noticeably straighten their backs and uncross their feet.

So self-assured was Mrs Wordsworth that she once allegedly offended Queen Victoria when the monarch entered her class to observe her teaching the Queen of Spain (Ripman, 1974). Mrs Wordsworth's loud 'shush' on hearing voices behind her resulted in the royal invitation to teach at the palace never being repeated. There were other teachers who benefited from occasional court patronage. The Bland family of father and daughters, for example, traded on a former royal connection in their newspaper advertisements over a number of years, while the Healey sisters, dancers at the King's Theatre, Copenhagen, held classes during the 1880s for children of the nobility at Stafford House.[15]

Although not regularly teaching a clientele as exclusive as Taglioni, the D'Egvilles, and Mrs Wordsworth, there were several professional dancers who regularly advertised in the quality press to attract Society and the upper bourgeoisie. During the 1870s, the *Times* carried several notices from both home-grown and foreign stage performers. Miss James of the Royal Opera offered daily lessons in which her pupils would have 'the great advantage of Miss James practising with them herself, which tends to rapid progress to those wholly unacquainted with dancing'.[16] The *cachet* of being taught by a French professional, formerly a *maître de ballet* at Her Majesty's Theatre, distinguished the services of Monsieur Emile Petit. Working with Madame Stephane Petit, he provided lessons in 'danse, bonne tenue, et calisteniques'.[17] Offering similar fare, but advertising in English, were 'les demoiselles Jay, daughters of the eminent Monsieur Alexandre (late of the Italian Opera)' who courted the 'nobility and gentry and principals of high-class schools' in the London districts of Kensington, South Hampstead, and Ealing, as well as in Brighton.[18] Teachers with this background sometimes taught more than movement suitable for the ball room. Fanny Wright, dancer with the Theatre Royal, Haymarket prepared 'ladies for stage dancing' as well as providing instruction in fashionable dances, and M. St Maine and his daughters of Drury Lane and Covent Garden taught fancy dances, elocution, and stage business, assuring clients of tuition in stage and ballroom dancing 'till perfect'.[19] During his residence in London during the 1870s, international ballet dancer Léon Espinosa, recently contracted with the Theatre Royal, Covent Garden and the opera houses of Saint Petersburg and Moscow, gave private lessons in deportment and fashionable dancing, the latter including 'the real mazurka as danced at the imperial courts'.[20]

High-class instructors targeted potential pupils through a language of servility and arcane courtesy. Phrases such as 'beg to inform' and 'have the honour to announce' peppered the advertisements along with insistent caveats that the service was for 'the children of gentlemen only' or 'exclusively for the families of the nobility and gentry'.[21] To signal exclusivity further, upmarket teachers habitually advertised fees in guineas rather than in the everyday parlance of shillings and pence, while a number of Society teachers eschewed public notice of their fees altogether, terms being available only on application. During the early 1870s, the standard rate for Society dance teachers was a guinea for four private lessons.[22] Expensive lessons obviously deterred the less wealthy, though high-class teachers deployed other socially restrictive devices, such as requesting references for new lady pupils or approving visiting cards before taking subscriptions from individuals to join dancing assemblies.[23]

Society teachers typically offered a variety of weekly sessions for adult beginners, as well as daily private lessons – especially in the Waltz – and Saturday classes for young ladies and children. Lessons in drawing room dancing became so popular among the upper bourgeoisie in London that a few more entrepreneurial teachers maintained elaborate schedules of classes and assemblies. The London Academy of Dancing, under the direction of Edward Humphrey, catered for all levels, grading proficiency and interest from A to H.[24] Course A was subdivided into four stages: the first where ladies and gentlemen were separately instructed in the steps, the second and third where they practised in combined classes, and finally the fourth where more advanced pupils progressed to the assemblies and balls held in the Cavendish Rooms of the London Academy. An annual subscription to this scheme cost a guinea and a half (one guinea for ladies) but pupils could enter at any point in the year. For those wanting shorter courses, a quarterly ticket was available for 15 shillings (half a guinea for ladies) which bought 20 separate classes, or a monthly ticket for seven shillings and sixpence (ladies five shillings) entitled the holder to eight classes. A single lesson plus participation in the assembly was available for two shillings and sixpence. Humphrey also offered discounts to groups, an annual family ticket for four costing two guineas for the classes in dancing, deportment, and callisthenics for 'ladies and juveniles'.

In addition to tuition in dancing and deportment, teachers, dependent on expertise, location, and inclination, offered a number of related services: they might run dance assemblies at their own academies, write prescriptive manuals on dancing, act as Master of Ceremonies at public dances, hire out their premises for social occasions, supply musicians for dances, compose dances (and occasionally music) for the ball or drawing room (and sometimes for the theatre), and instruct new or existing members of the profession in their art.

Several London-based teachers such as Leonora Geary, Henri Dacunha, Mrs Henderson, Edward Humphrey, and Edward Lawson published guides to the ball room, sometimes on an annual basis, so that their pupils and other purchasers could keep up with fashion.[25] These guides usually opened with an address to pupils, especially the aristocracy and gentry, followed by a short, mostly regurgitated, introduction on dance history and the value of dancing to health and social life. This then gave way to the main content of the book which was composed of fairly rudimentary descriptions of the various dances current in the ball room, notated in word and diagram. More considered distillations of knowledge and experience appeared from the 1890s in specialist articles by dancing masters Robert Crompton, Charles D'Albert, and to a lesser extent, Louis D'Egville in the new professional journals. The most prolific writer on dance, teacher Edward Scott aimed at a more ambitious appreciation, publishing numerous books on the technique and history of dancing, as well as becoming a regular contributor to Richardson's second series of the *Dancing Times*.

Another mode of income was the composition of new dances for the Society drawing room. As print communication expanded, an increasing number appeared each year and the more successful teachers travelled to impart their new choreographies to members of the profession. Edouard LeBlanc's *La Nationale*, Robert Crompton's *Iolanthe*, and Walter Humphrey's *Hussars* enjoyed limited circulation within Society,[26] but it was not an especially lucrative aspect of their trade. As Scott woefully revealed years later, despite the relative popularity of his own invention, the *Chorolistha* for which he composed both music and choreography, the dance earned him only £300 over several decades.[27]

For centuries, the correct execution of dancing and deportment within Society had lain beyond the reach of autodidactism, but in the eyes of many teachers the unchallenging American dances of the 1890s posed a potential threat to the future of the pedagogic profession. The repertoire was quickly learned by those already versed in Victorian ball room technique, and even those with little experience might venture imitation on the dance floor. Easy dances did not require lessons from a professional; teachers, particularly those lacking royal patronage, were anxious that their livelihood was in peril.

8
Temples of Terpsichore

> to endeavour to elevate the dancing profession, and to
> raise the standard of ability of its members.
>
> *Dancing*, 8 June 1891, p. 10

Dancing schools were occasionally advertised for sale, mostly on the death or retirement of the owner. Details of location or ownership were rarely cited, no doubt to minimize unease among the existing clientele. Often the school was of long standing, as for example that advertised in the *Times* in 1890, which after 41 years became available to a 'young person' with £300 to enter a partnership. In general, however, turnover in the more reputable schools was limited.[1] Teachers generally enjoyed longevity in their careers before handing on the business to family members or to long-term assistant teachers whom they had often schooled themselves.

The traditional training grounds for high-class teachers of dancing and deportment were the institutions of the family and the stage which, as in the case of the D'Egville Michau, Gilmer, and Soutten families were often intertwined.[2] For many intending teachers, however, a well-trodden route was the articled pupil system. Practised across a range of trades and services in Britain, the articled pupil system contracted a young person to an apprenticeship with a senior practitioner who offered tuition, experience, and occasionally board and lodgings. These facilities were supplied in return for money, assistance with teaching in the school, and sometimes duties around the home. Actual copies of contracts between a social dancing teacher and articled pupil have yet to come to light; evidence of their existence and detail rests mainly on advertisements, fleshed out by occasional references in biographical material, or in later articles in professional journals. There is also limited comparable information from the music profession. In the eighteenth and earlier nineteenth centuries, many teachers were expert in both music and dance, but by the later nineteenth century, such pedagogic breadth was more infrequent, lingering longest among the older families who passed their musical skills down the generations.[3]

Census returns identify assistants sometimes as visitors to the teacher's home, but also as residential trainees. Once judged expert by their mentor, the fledgling teacher could be engaged as an employee, if the size and success of the school merited an extra position. The majority of trainees and assistant teachers by the late nineteenth century were young women. Madame Adelaide, daughter of the celebrated Madame Michau, provided lodging and training to at least three daughters of the Walsh family. In 1901, Ernest Gilmer, son of professional opera ballet dancer James Gilmer, housed four articled pupils, together with a non-family assistant teacher, all female. In a rather more intimate arrangement, Patience Alice Parker, assistant teacher to the already married Edward Scott and resident at his home and studio in Hove, became the mother of his third child and, much later, his second wife.[4]

The newly qualified could seek a position as assistant teacher with another school. Successful teachers with an established reputation and large clientele were able to attract, and had need of, more assistant instructors to cope with the workload, particularly for teaching classes out of town. In 1872 Madame Adelaide advertised the availability of her own pupils to teach in the country, a practice similarly followed by Madame Stainton Taylor of the South Kensington School of Dancing.[5] Advertisements for assistant teachers sometimes stipulated existing skills. In 1880, Madame D'Egville Michau of Brighton, required a 'good pianiste', aged about 22 years for a position as 'resident assistant'. It seems as if the appointment was unsatisfactory as the following year a renewed advert stipulates that the applicant 'understands something of the profession ... must be ladylike in manner and appearance, play the piano well, and give good references'.[6] Assistant teachers could succeed to the whole business on the death or retirement of their former mentor, especially in cases where there were no offspring to take over the school, or else the children's career plans formed a different trajectory from that of their parents. Daughters, for example, might leave the dancing profession on marriage, to attain the coveted middle-class status of a non-working wife. Increasingly, too, sons turned away from the dancing studio towards alternative careers, often as white collar workers in offices.[7]

Directories and census returns in the London area indicate a rise in the number of dance teachers towards the end of the century, in part to cater for the burgeoning and increasingly affluent middle classes of the city's population. Many of the neophyte dance teachers left the school of their training to set up business on their own, often advertising their credentials by referring to their former tutors. Courtesy and business acumen suggested that the newcomer did not encroach upon the catchment area of their previous instructor. During the 1890s, there were frequent complaints about ill-qualified newcomers moving nearby to set up in opposition to a long-established school; indeed, among the properly qualified, some new teachers poached their own mentors' pupils. There was even concern about potential competition within family dynasties. James Paul Michau's will of 1877 stipulates that his daughter must not teach dancing within 50 miles of Brighton town hall, in order to protect the livelihood of his only son to whom he bequeathed his school. As late as 1918, the *Dancing Times* suggested that established teachers took recourse to the law in order to prevent neighbouring competition from recent graduates, and recommended a minimum of 15 miles distance over a period of three years.[8]

Other threats to the established teacher came from the cheaper priced lessons offered by charlatan competitors. 'Only those desiring the best instruction, and having the good sense to know that it is more advantageous than cheap lessons, need trouble to call' pronounced high-class dancing master Edward Scott who frequently condemned the techniques and knowledge base of provincial and poorly trained teachers.[9] Unlike music pedagogy which had become professionalized through institutions such as the Royal Academy of Music, there was no nationally agreed system of certification for dancing teachers. This situation was much lamented by London dancing master Robert Crompton who mounted a campaign through his journal *Dancing* to mobilize his colleagues towards a more professionalized service and status (Buckland, 2007). Too often, he claimed, new teachers began without the necessary years of training and supervised practice, thus spoiling the reputation of the profession overall, engendering aesthetic damage to the standards of dancing in the ballroom, and potentially inflicting physical injury to their pupils when training them in the more demanding technical requirements for the stage. Well-known teachers such as Humphrey at the London Academy of Dancing, as well as Crompton at his West End base, offered certificated courses, but exactly what each teacher offered and how the provision compared are impossible to judge.[10] Credibility continued to rest on the reputation and credentials of individuals, not on the agreed criteria of any national institution, until the early twentieth century.

Protecting the profession

Although dance teachers typically enjoyed longevity and a healthy constitution, their livelihoods were potentially at risk from physical injury, poor health, and downturns in the market. Various occupational groups since the eighteenth century had taken the precaution of forming friendly and benefit societies to insure against such risks and to protect the vulnerable within their ranks. A growing number had united to defend the standards of their activities against poorly qualified newcomers and regulated entry to their profession through the institution of courses and examinations at national level. This widespread move towards professionalization through self-regulation was a constituent feature of the expanding Victorian middle classes, effecting a shift away from the traditional network of familial and social relations towards a system based upon paper accreditation. Practice and personal testimonials now counted less than the certificate awarded by a centralized organizational structure of committees and examination boards, often, as in the cases of the Royal College of Music, the Royal Academy of Music, and the Royal College of Art, with national headquarters of instruction based in the capital.[11]

Dance pedagogy was slow to follow suit, both with respect to the emergence of insurance societies and the establishment of a professional society to uphold standards in the public interest and that of their members. There had been abortive attempts since the eighteenth century to unite, but the highly individualized and competitive nature of the occupation tended to mitigate against communal activity. By the very end of the nineteenth century, however, complaints about the status of dance teachers, well rehearsed in the previous century, had gained new prominence. Correspondence and editorial commentary in *Dancing*, in *The Dancing Times*, and more broadly in the Society press drew attention to a complex of factors that now threatened the profession of dancing teachers: widespread tolerance of poor dancing in Society circles; a growing inclination towards an easier repertoire, as evidenced in American dances such as the *Washington Post* and the Two-Step; the contraction of peripatetic work in schools as competitive outdoor sports and gymnastics gained ground in the curriculum, and the new vigilance in operating the licensing laws. The academies of dancing teachers were subject to the mid-eighteenth-century Disorderly Houses Act (Act 25 Geo.II, c. 36) whereby any premises for public dancing required a licence. From 1888, applications for such licences were dealt with by the metropolitan authorities, some of whose members exercised moral as well as public order concerns.[12] The puritanical element among these largely middle-class urban boards viewed public dancing with suspicion as a potential site for theft, drunkenness, and prostitution. Coupled with new legislation to protect the public from fire and building hazards, the licensing laws proved a considerable barrier to dancing instructors' livelihoods. As a consequence, a number of long-established teachers, such as Thomas Upton and Francis Piaggio, were prosecuted for failing to procure the necessary licence.[13] The majority of teachers affected by these licensing laws catered for the mid-to-lower middle classes, rather than members of high Society who could gather in large private houses to dance with total impunity from the law: the licensing laws protected the moneyed, but often prevented the ordinary person from enjoying dancing as an innocent pastime.[14]

It was in this context that the initiatives towards a national organization of dancing teachers in England became successful when the British Association of Teachers of Dancing (BATD) was founded in 1892. The BATD grew from its initial core of 24 members to 120 by 1897, though its upwards trajectory became chequered by internal dissent and resignation, leading to the formation of other societies with similar aims in the early 1900s.[15] The higher echelons of the dance-teaching profession, however, remained aloof from such ventures. Secure in their patronage from courtly circles, they felt no need of the protective force of institutional affiliation. Pleas for the involvement of the Society teachers to legitimize and add prestige to association fell on deaf ears. The BATD nonetheless continued to grow apace, celebrating its centenary in 1992, as the oldest national organization of dancing teachers in Britain. The organization was registered as a friendly society in 1896 and remained the only dance organization in the twentieth century to offer such support to its subscribers. Every year its members held a convention to discuss matters of concern to the profession and also to hold competitions for the best social dance composition.[16]

The increasing feminization of dance pedagogy

Prior to the late-nineteenth century, the majority of female teachers had appeared in a familial role as wife or daughter to the dancing master. Notable examples include the husband and wife teams of Michau, Sheridan Lings, Henderson and Wynman, and the daughters of Dachuna, Bland, LeBlanc, and Henderson.[17] Single female teachers, however, were not exceptional. To the roll call of the famous such as Marie Taglioni, the former English ballet dancer Madame Soutten, and Society teacher

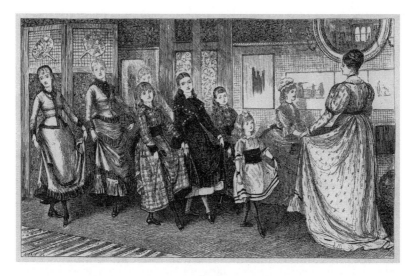

Figure 8.1 Dancing Class c. 1880 (George du Maurier)

Miss Leonora Geary, can be added the various prominent female members of the Michau D'Egville family – Isabel Michau, Madame Adelaide, and Caroline D'Egville Michau – as well as Miss Cornelia Vincent, Miss Elizabeth Garratt, Madame Stainton Taylor, and, not forgetting the celebrated Mrs Wordsworth. By the late 1890s and early 1900s, however, there was a different trend discernible in the increasing number of female assistants training for a career in dance pedagogy, often without any stage or family connections to the profession (see Figure 8.1).

The appearance of this new female contingent, many of whom tended to specialize in fancy dances, did not go uncriticized by Edward Scott. In his opinion, they merely provided a service for gullible undiscerning parents who wanted their children to learn fashionable dances as quickly and as showily as possible. Scott warned of the dangers of the move towards large classes in which novices were placed at the back where they could not see the teacher, their view obstructed by specially trained pupils placed in the front rows 'merely to make a pretty and alluring show'.[18] The custom of positioning a more proficient dancer at the front of the class for others to copy had precedence. Nonetheless there was a considerable distinction between the small groups of Society teachers such as Taglioni and D'Egville, whose teaching was conditioned both by the size of home premises and a royal command to maintain an exclusive clientele, and the larger class sizes of fashionable female teachers in the 1890s. By then, some female Society teachers, such as Madame Stainton Taylor and Elizabeth Garratt, as well as Mrs Wordsworth, were hiring large public spaces such as Queens Gate Hall in Kensington and Kensington Town Hall (built 1880) to meet the demand for children's and young ladies' classes.[19]

In spite of her sense of social exclusivity, Mrs Wordsworth capitalized upon the situation, profiting from her cultural cachet as teacher to aristocracy and the occasional royal, as well as oft-reported contributor to numerous fashionable charitable events at which her privileged young clientele performed. She rejected the stage as a legitimate destination for her pupils, condemning a theatrical career as a morally dubious enterprise. Instead, Mrs Wordsworth stressed the social and healthy benefits of dancing and physical culture.[20] As teacher of the rich and royal, her system signalled social approval, and wealthy parents were anxious to include their child in the dancing classes of the social elite. Indeed, even if parents were unable to acquire direct tuition for their offspring in the classes of the doyenne herself, such was the teacher's fame that many a snobbish client was proud to claim a genealogy of instruction through one of her many pupil teachers (Nickalls, 1958).

Cannily, Mrs Wordsworth had taken the existing articled pupil system, expanded and accelerated it, and devised a scheme of tuition that could be replicated by her young female teachers up and down the country. Former trainee Olive Ripman recalled how, as one of 12–14 middle-class girls seeking a career in dance teaching (circa 1907), she lodged in a house next to Queensberry Hall in South Kensington where Mrs Wordsworth maintained her headquarters with the help of a secretary. Travelling by train four days a week from her Surrey home, 'Wordy' as her trainees referred to her, rarely taught a whole lesson. Her army of assistant and student teachers shouldered this responsibility. Any student who showed aptitude in dancing was soon deployed as a demonstrator and helper to senior teachers in various venues across London. This practice constituted the apprentice teachers' principal experience of pedagogic training, their role in class being

> to keep the lines straight, help the "flounderers", act as the odd partner and so on. The teacher taking the class just sailed about the room giving commands and calling "Stand", "Go", "Next", and "By yourself." She always wore a long dress and train, and spent most of the time putting on gloves or taking them off.
>
> (Ripman, 1974, p. 639)

When not assisting, student teachers participated in the general classes which never deviated in structure and content: first of all, skipping using ropes, then club swinging, marching in formation around the room in couples, arm exercises while kneeling on one knee, steps (ballet-based such as coupés, ballonnés, and related Highland dancing movements such as reel steps), a fancy dance specially composed for each term and round dancing. The latter, before commencing which all pupils drew on mittens in imitation of the gloved Society dancers, began with the Galop, then Polka, Waltz, the *Barn Dance*, and, if time permitted, the *Washington Post*. The class concluded with a march round in a column formation and curtsey.

In addition to this unvarying fare, student teachers joined in classes in fencing, Swedish drill and gymnastics, elocution, skirt dancing, and Highland dancing, the latter examined by specialists. The course of instruction at Mrs Wordsworth's academy lasted two years and was followed by summer term sessions during which the teachers instructed one another in 'anything that they had picked up during the year' (Ripman, 1974, p. 639). Ripman describes a heavy schedule of travelling and teaching across the south-east of England as one of the many Edwardian pupil teachers trained under the Wordsworth system. In spite of its hardships, restrictions, and lack of exposure to theatrical dance training, she nonetheless appears indebted to the experience that immediate immersion in teaching practice brought to her future career as a very successful teacher of dancing.

Ripman is typical of the new wave of young middle-class women in dance pedagogy and whose numbers would steadily increase. Dance pedagogy was judged to be a suitably ladylike profession, and potentially lucrative (even promising higher social mobility), especially if the trainee instructor were to be apprenticed to an established teacher with a high-ranking clientele. The reputable teacher of deportment and drawing room dances Miss Vincent, when interviewed in 1911 suggested that the potential income compared 'quite favourably with their learned sisters' in the profession of school teachers. Indeed, she revealed, the more successful dancing teachers could command annual salaries of up to four figures.[21]

Alongside ideological factors that aligned women with dancing (see Chapters 9 and 10), there were wider social, economic, and demographic developments at the end of the century that contributed to the growing feminization of the profession. Demanding greater equality and opportunity in their lives, respectable career options for women by the 1890s had expanded beyond the established prospects of wife or governess.

Employed as journalists, school teachers, clerks, and typists, some middle-class women, including indeed a few of genteel lineage, aspired to a more high profile and glamorous employment in the theatre or in the new role of fashion model (see Chapter 10). The desire to work was also in many cases governed by necessity. In late nineteenth-century Britain, birth and survival rates for females far outnumbered those of males, reducing the pool of eligible young bachelors. Furthermore, bourgeois men tended to delay taking on the social and financial responsibilities of husband and father until their late twenties and early thirties, while the expense of dowries and keeping women at home were often beyond the purse of many families.[22] Dance pedagogy appeared as a suitably genteel occupation for middle-class young women; while those secure in Society or young enough to entertain social ambitions, continued to receive instruction in good deportment and the basic ball room repertoire, dreaming of a debut at a glittering ball and of being presented at court.

9
The Fashioning of Ladies

> If a girl is to go into society, give her the advantage of
> being taught to move like a lady.
>> Madame D'Egville Michau, *Treatise on
>> Deportment, Dancing, and Physical Education
>> for Young Ladies*, 1861, p. 32

The socialization of aristocratic Victorian women inherited much from eighteenth-century practice and discourse. Fashioned as wife, mother, and hostess, an upper-class woman's appearance, behaviour and duty to Society remained paramount. Although the posture and movement of both men and women, born to the ranks of royalty and aristocracy, were expected to be characterized by elegance, absence of affectation and exaggeration, ease, poise, and grace, it was this latter quality of grace that was especially prized for females. Dancing in the ball room and in the drawing room provided opportunity for the leisured single young woman to make a quiet and tasteful exhibition of her embodiment of gracefulness, both as an aesthetic pleasure for all onlookers and, more importantly, as an attraction to procure a marriage partner.

The aristocratic ideals of gentle and graceful dignity of person were epitomized in the person of the gentlewoman or *lady*; for it was she who was considered the touchstone and keeper of civilization. Her role was to act as a civilizing force to temper the supposedly more brutish tendencies of men. As Lady Violet Greville (1892, pp. 270–1) concluded in her advisory manual:

[T]he work of the Gentlewoman in Society is to purify, and refine, and to elevate; to teach modesty and grace and truth; to set an example of fine manners; to impose the laws of order and decorum; and to place before man an Ideal of unpurchasable Beauty and Dignity which he may learn to love, reverence, and imitate.

It was incumbent upon ladies to present such an ideal in the ball room. As a growing number of men eschewed the dance floor during the late Victorian period, dancing and gracefulness became ever more strongly associated with perceptions of idealized femininity. Growing prosperity and social aspiration prompted many a middle-class family to bring up their daughters as ladies in manner and, hopefully through later marriage, turn into ladies in status. Becoming 'ladylike' was a potential ticket to being a genuine lady.

At the very time that Violet Greville was advocating and extolling the virtues of ladylike behaviour, a number of upper-class young women were turning their backs against such a limiting and impossible role, to the shock and horror of the stalwarts of Society. Types of middle- and upper-class women other than 'the lady' had become recognized in society, notably the keen sportswoman, the blue-stocking intellectual, and by the mid 1890s, the independent New Woman, reputed to be more mannish in appearance and behaviour than her opposite sex and thus most criticized by conservatives who feared upset of the biological and social order (Crow, 1971; Vicinus, 1972, 1977, 1985; Heilmann, 1998). In spite of the growth and increasing acceptance of alternative lifestyles for middle- and upper-class women in the 1890s, however, the cultural ideal of 'the lady' remained resilient. A lady was the true guardian of moral values and social etiquette within the bourgeois cult of gentility, imitating the higher echelons of Society and the court circle.

Moving as a lady

Codified bodily inscriptions of gender, occupation, and social status to signal the elite had long been part of the civilizing process in European society (Elias, 1978; Bourdieu, 1984). For women, there was an added moral dimension. An aristocratic woman, or indeed one of a reputable family, was identifiable through an unaffected display of modesty, in expected contrast to her less respected sisters, notably a lower-class female or, worse still, a prostitute. Social proxemics and bodily control distinguished the woman of breeding, her social and moral standing evidenced in her controlled access to physical space, her narrow personal kinesphere, her limited movement dynamics, and her constrained spatial relationships with the opposite sex. Upper-class women never appeared alone in public; they did not call attention to themselves either through occupying a large amount of space, or through using quick and forceful movement; and they preserved a guarded bodily distance in all public social interactions with men, even if they were close friends or family members.

Moreover, the posture and gait of a woman of breeding were distinct from those of a man. In the nineteenth century, long-standing culturally gendered distinctions were consolidated, largely underpinned by new research into human anatomy and by the development of physiology as a science that established biology as the single factor in determining gender (Gallagher and Laqueur, 1987). Whereas gender in the eighteenth century had been largely regarded as a process of socialization, the Victorians perceived masculinity and femininity to be biologically polar essences. According to this world view, which was supported by contemporary philosophical, religious, and educational discourse, Nature had created man and woman as different but complementary. For the educated Victorian, men were naturally strong, active, and rational, whereas women were weak, passive, and emotional. Such contrastive roles were expected to be played out socially and physically.

A lady's pace was to be narrower than that of a man, her energy levels lower, her foot movements closer to the floor, her legs never to be lifted or kicked, her feet daintily pointed and her arm movements rounded, and controlled, never flung or outstretched, or swung when walking. Doyenne of courtly etiquette Marie Taglioni complained that it 'made her ill to see women swing their arms like men' (Rolfe). Ladies never ran in the streets, or indeed in any social situation, nor were they to indulge in physical actions that might cause them to become hot and uncomfortable. In everyday interactions, whenever a lady re-orientated her gaze or direction, she was expected to initiate the change of focus by using her head with 'a snakelike movement' (Rolfe) never with her whole body, so that she moved with sinuous grace. In the ball room, the women's dance steps, mirroring or reversing those of her partner were smaller and less energetic. Throughout all her actions, the containment of physicality was essential to the look of a lady, as enshrined in the contemporary maxim, 'horses sweat, men perspire, ladies glow'. The lady should never reveal any physical exertion or clumsiness in bodily etiquette, even though the elaborate moves of greeting and leave-taking required much greater practice and control than the simple acknowledging bow of the late Victorian gentleman.

Society ladies at court

The dictates of ladylike movement looked back to earlier times when ballet and royalty shared a closer aesthetic. In the 1870s, Marie Taglioni's graceful and measured deportment remained to be much admired by the Queen and the court inner circle as a model of decorum for aristocratic women, even though the young generation found it far too theatrical for polite modern tastes. When the elderly ballerina retired backwards out of a room, she would execute a half curtsey while throwing 'un regard circulaire' to the assembled company before seemingly 'melting' through the door (Rolfe). Silent, graceful movement continued to be viewed as evidence of ladylike behaviour for later generations, but exaggerated movement in daily interaction had been replaced by a calm simplicity of movement to reflect the 'English' character which was perceived to be honest, direct, and lacking in unnecessary gesticular action.[1] Quieter and less fussy than that of her continental counterparts, the deportment of an Englishwoman was celebrated as expressive of the national psyche. Her even, noiseless gliding along the floor contrasted with the short, mincing steps of fashionable French women. Regarded as naturally calm and elegant, though obviously trained to be such, the ladies of the British Empire, like their husbands, were ideally calm, ordered, and unflappable in every situation, their regal posture and measured locomotion reflecting their innate ability to rule over other classes and races.

Nowhere was the performance of an aristocratic English mien and knowledge of bodily etiquette more important for a woman than when presented at the British court. For a woman to enter into full Society life, presentation to the Queen in the ritual known as Her Majesty's Drawing Room was mandatory (Armytage, 1883). Not only might the initiate then be invited to state balls (though this was not an automatic privilege) but she might also attend functions at other European royal courts. It was in these lengthy Drawing Rooms held each year during the Season that the neophyte's skills in graceful, controlled movement were tested. Each year London-based deportment specialists tutored aristocratic girls from the country, American socialites, and the more socially successful of the *nouveaux riches* in the necessary carriage and etiquette. Learning how to glide slowly and smoothly, to manage the long train, to carry gloves, a fan and flowers, and to execute the deep curtsey before the monarch while kissing her hand could prove especially tricky for a nervous young woman.[2] By the 1870s, the deep curtsey before social superiors in daily interaction had become outmoded, although as the favoured pupil of Marie Taglioni, young Margaret Rolfe could not escape the demands of a less fashionable but more polite age. She dreaded street encounters with her teacher and grandmother on account of the older women's stipulation that she make at least two deep curtseys to each of them. Rolfe was ever fearful of 'making an exhibition of myself in the street' and complained that the deep curtsey 'took an eternity, with eyelids lowered, and then slowly raised'. Retained in court ritual, the proper execution of the deep curtsey proved particularly daunting for the debutante for it demanded control, balance, and carefully sustained timing:

> First, you draw back the right foot, getting it straight behind the other, and down you go, as far as the suppleness of your limbs will permit, coming up to the "recover" with all the weight on the right foot, and the left pointed out most daintily.
>
> (Humphry, 1897b, p. 7)

In preparation for the London Season, anxious women practised these deep curtseys and the gliding, slow walk in front of their deportment mentors and fellow pupils. Balancing books on their heads to cultivate poise, they rehearsed the ceremony, tablecloths wrapped around their waists and draped over their arms to emulate the train. Many a debutante was haunted by fears of hitting her nose on the Queen's hand as she kissed the royal person, of treading on the train of the woman in front, and of over-balancing in the curtsey. Once safely past the Queen, she still had to curtsey deeply to each member of the royal family before a page swept the long train over her arm as the signal to move on. Earlier in the century, the statelier and comparatively sparsely attended Drawing Rooms had allowed time for a well-spaced procession and for the performance of slow, deep curtseys. Not so in Rolfe's day: at her own somewhat more crowded court presentation, she 'entirely stopped the procession and had to finish up with half curtseys. If everyone had curtsied "à la Taglioni" the court would have lasted a week'. No wonder that Princess May, later to become Queen Mary, then Rolfe's classmate in Taglioni's dancing and deportment lessons, expressed relief that her own royal position exempted her from this ordeal (see Figure 9.1).

Fashioning the body of a lady

The fashioning of a lady's body and movement owed much to the corsetière and dressmaker as well as to her peer group and dancing and deportment instructors. The ideal body shape for upper-class women was largely constructed by corsets which, as an undergarment once worn by both sexes for support and warmth of the torso, had by the nineteenth century become a highly gendered item of clothing which shaped the female body into a rigid and structured ideal of bodily femininity (Summers, 2003). The late Victorian corset created an extreme hourglass

100

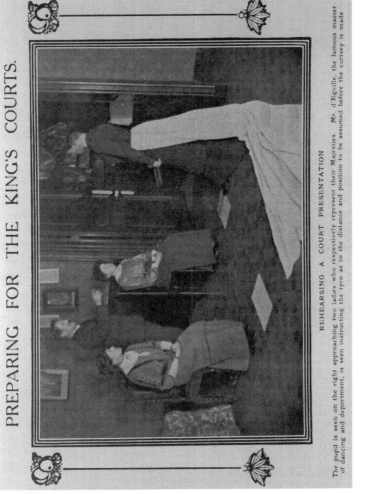

Figure 9.1 Preparing for the King's Courts, *The Tatler*, 18 January 1911

figure, the waist constricted by tight lacing to an exceptionally narrow circumference of around 18–20 inches. Full breasts, curvaceous hips, and an artificially attained girlish waist signalled the mature, sexually experienced woman, the ideal Society hostess of the inner court circle, as exemplified in the figures of the Prince of Wales's married and high status mistresses, Lilly Langtry and Alice Keppel.

Dancing teachers, physical educationalists, moralists, health reformers, rational dress advocates and female emancipators conducted long and high profile campaigns against the excesses of the fashionable corset as it compressed the lower ribs and prevented proper breathing. But a preference for unfettered garments that might enable freedom of movement and improve female health, instead of following the latest fashions, was slow to infiltrate the aristocratic feminine consciousness and their bourgeois imitators. All Victorian women wore corsets, though of variable quality and age, including women who worked in the fields, factories, and in service. The expensive services of a corsetière for the new season's well-boned, bespoke garment, available only to the wealthy, were yet another means of displaying gendered wealth and status. The aristocratic female body was made rigidly upright, incapable of moving quickly or bending inelegantly, for it did not need to; the ideal aristocratic feminine form was a still, contained, and decorative figure. The ample proportions of the well-fed, soft, and rounded female body, undefined by the muscles of hard labour or made thin by the restricted diet of poverty, exhibited the leisured existence of its wearer.

The fashionable corset forced the wearer's breasts upwards which, in the décolleté gowns of the ballroom, rendered women even more sexually alluring, especially when they panted in quick shallow breaths after a fast Waltz drew to a close. Much of the complaint against the hazards of waltzing for young women came from those of a more puritanical persuasion who had little time for the idle pastimes of Society. Moral reformers of an evangelical hue had penned numerous tracts on the proper conduct of young women in the early nineteenth century, a vein of which flowed through into the latter part of Victoria's reign.[3] Puritanical clergy frequently expressed concern for the health of young women in fashionably tight clothes, exposing bare shoulders in the evening air, becoming overheated and dizzy in the Waltz and breathing gas and candle fumes in the overcrowded balls and drawing rooms, although the criticism amounted to nothing like the volume and sense of moral panic that raged in the more puritanical United States (Wagner, 1997). Not surprisingly, the results of very tight lacing by ladies of fashion contributed to the widespread belief that hysteria, often brought on by hyperventilation, was a natural female disposition. Tales of women being cut from their corsets after fainting while dancing abound, the exceptionally plump but small-waisted Countess of Erne reputedly suffering this ignominious fate in the middle of a Kitchen Lancers (Stewart, 1938).

Female movement was further limited by the long-trained skirt worn with an overskirt for evening dress, a shape which developed into a tight sheath in the late 1870s (Cunnington and Cunnington, 1966). The next decade saw an even longer train and the return of the bustle, which projected sharply out from the verticality of the spine, not only encumbering rapid movement on account of the sheer size of the bustle, but also because of the uncomfortable weight of extra fabric and steel hoops. Scott (1887b, p. 57) had no doubt that such 'exaggerated extension is inelegant and vulgar', resembling, he jibed, the buttocks of the 'Hottentot Venus' and contradicting the Hogarthian 'line of beauty'. A former lithographer and devotee of art, Scott drew his own aesthetic appreciation of the female form from Hellenic principles. His ideal female body was the Venus de Milo, sculptured as if draped with naturally falling folds of cloth and unrestricted by the excessive control of voguish attire. Although, like most of his contemporaries, Scott allowed for the wearing of supportive undergarments, it was the extremes of conical waists and large posteriors, conceived as aesthetically pleasing to the eye of fashion, that were antithetical to his notion of civilization. Such distortions of the human frame and the discomfort endured by the wearer he considered to be comparable with the practices of non-European peoples whose customary re-shapings of the human body were, he pronounced, the result of ignorance.

Scott was not alone in aligning dress, health, and nature as markers of civilization. Whereas artifice had once distinguished civilization in the eighteenth century, during the Victorian period, recourse to the 'natural' had increasingly been accorded greater value by doctors and education-alists writing on the cultivation of the healthy human body. A number of the various rational dress organizations that drew greater support from the 1880s onwards (Newton, 1974; Wilson, 2003) were nonetheless unwilling to sacrifice cultural concepts of grace and beauty while cloth-ing the female form. Any garment that suggested masculine habits such as the infamous bloomers worn for cycling was ridiculed in the press in spite of the practicality of such attire for the activity. Any hint of cross-dressing in the social (but not the popular stage) arena or exposure of the lower limbs and naked flesh was at the very least likely to summon ref-erence to fictitious moral guardian Mrs Grundy who patrolled Victorian sensibilities of decency and order.

Dress reformers' efforts to persuade stylish women to relinquish their restrictive and uncomfortable clothing took time; other influential cultural, political, and economic shifts in society occurred before more freedom of movement and consequent better health prospects for women were secured. Specially designed clothing to pursue physical activities such as walking, golf, tennis, cycling and for the very rich, riding and shooting, appeared late in the century. For social dancing, however, an activity in the realm of the ultra fashionable, Parisian fashion designers continued to hold sway. A ball gown remained the most elaborate mode of dress whereby a woman might display herself publicly to her peers at her most beautiful and desirable. The fact that the design of the garment often ran counter to the idea of moving easily and gracefully was irrelevant.

Fashionable footwear further hampered comfortable and graceful dancing. During the 1880s, the 'preposterous high-heeled, pointed French boots' were condemned by Scott (1887b, p. 47) as causing unnecessary muscular strain and fatigue. Throwing the weight too far forwards and crushing the toes, these boots also forced their wearers to walk with bent knees and the percussive effect of placing the whole foot on the floor when walking threatened damage to the spine. Such habits of a resultant 'undignified gait' were transferred to the ball room, the high heels of the 1890s slipper for evening wear (Cunnington and Cunnington, 1966) adding to the discomfort. Nonetheless, by the 1890s, there was growing acceptance that women were more desirable and useful to society if physically active. There was a shift towards a female body that was tall and healthy, but paradoxically this physical ideal was often achieved through donning exceptionally tight corsets and high heels. The contradictions and tensions in this decade with respect to the role and image of women are captured in this paradox and typified the figures of the modern New Woman versus the Society woman of fashion.

A lady's physical education

For the prosperous middle class, an alternative education lay in the genteel girls' boarding schools that sprang up from the end of the eighteenth century offering 'few academic pretensions and many social ones' (Vicinus, 1985, p. 165). Until the closing decades of Victoria's reign, these establishments remained the principal means of education for well-to-do young women. Run principally by spinsters and widows, the schools focused on what were considered to be social accomplishments for young ladies – playing the piano, needlework, French, dancing, and deportment.

Caroline D'Egville Michau's treatise of 1861 on physical education and deportment for young ladies exemplifies Victorian expectations. Whereas boys' physical activities were competitive and outdoor in nature, the girls pursued dancing and skipping, both of which were mostly conducted indoors. The socialization of middle- and upper-class girls into exhibiting quieter, less boisterous behaviour normally began at the age of six or seven. At this age, they began to walk with their governess rather than play in the open air or nursery. From the age of ten, the loose-fitting foundation garment, tellingly known as 'stays', was replaced by the boned corset. After the age of 12, girls rarely ran or skipped as such movements were not considered proper for a young lady. Excessive hours spent reading in school rooms might develop crooked or hunched backs which, as well as being unhealthy, were aesthetically undesirable. By the 1840s, gentle callisthenics had replaced the eighteenth-century custom of fastening a board to the back to keep the spine upright and contraptions to force the feet outwards to cultivate an aristocratic gait had been abandoned.

There was a considerable body of public opinion by the 1870s, much of it influenced by philosopher and sociologist Herbert Spencer's writings on education (1861), to address the impoverished mental and physical diet offered to well-to-do young ladies (see, for example, Pascoe, 1879). Attempts at reform were largely tied to the Victorian obsession with preserving and promoting good health, not just for the well-being of the individual and family, but also of nation and empire. Dancing teachers tended to repeat the ideas of their eighteenth-century predecessors, impressing upon their audience the social as well as physical benefits of dancing for women:

> I consider it of great importance for a Lady to cultivate those accomplishments by which her appearance and form are improved ... the happiness, good temper and usefulness of women depend in a vast degree upon the amount of health they enjoy.
>
> (LeBlanc, [1883], pp. 5–6, 8)

Spencer's progressive ideas on physical education promoted better physical development for young women, but even so, his highly influential form of social Darwinism (see Dyhouse, 1976) continued to impede the full intellectual development of women. His ideas on the female role in society were firmly of his time and sex. Not unsurprisingly, the deeply conservative Scott concurred with Spencer's dislike of the blue stocking as a suitable role model for young women, (1911, p. 95) and recommended that

> [i]f parents wish to make their daughters really attractive, they cannot do better than have them properly instructed in the art of ornamental dancing. When thus employed, a graceful and beautiful girl is seen at her very best, and appears infinitely more charming than she would if making a display of erudition.

The type of physical exercise considered suitable for a lady remained an issue in developing healthy – or hygienic in nineteenth-century parlance – young women to become respectable wives and mothers. As the more physically delicate sex, women, Victorians believed, along with very young boys, should undertake only gentle exercise to develop strong lungs and a straight spine. Taglioni devoted a considerable part of her lessons to exercises rather than to dancing, much to Margaret Rolfe's disappointment. Amid the interminable *ronds de jambes*, there was a kneeling exercise which necessitated 'continual expense' in replacing stockings:

> It was <u>very</u> easy to do, but I was the only one who could do it, because when rising or bending back you were not allowed to help oneself with the hands or shoulder-blades and had to rise or sink <u>very slowly</u> [double underlining in original] using only the back. The knees had to be close together ... the hands were kept crossed on the breast <u>all</u> the time.

Mrs Wordsworth's pupil Olive Ripman (1974, p. 581) recalled that after their callisthenic exercises:

> we did our spot of dancing. Strictly fancy – starting with arm exercises done for some reason with a flower in one hand, and kneeling on one knee. Then Steps! Oh those steps (probably handed down from French emigrés who taught Court dancing but, as performed by us, quite unrecognisable).

Many high-class dancing teachers were united in opposition to the rise of gymnastics as appropriate exercise for women. Such types of physical exercise were judged to inhibit gracefulness and to develop elements of masculinity in the female physique. Dancing and deportment teachers should be 'training future ladies, not Amazons' (D'Egville Michau, 1861, p. 51) The fear was that gymnastics might 'coarsen' the bodily appearance of a lady and any potential comparison with the body of a manual labourer was to be avoided at all costs. *Cassells Household Guide* advised its middle-class readers to favour callisthenics over gymnastics for young women

> as gymnastics cause a gradual increase in the strength and aptitude of every part of the human frame, so also calisthenics [*sic*] affect to bring about the same development of limbs and muscles, the same acquisition of health and vigour, by gentle means, imparting at the same time a grace not to be acquired in the gymnasium.
>
> ([c. 1880], vol. 1, p. 25)

Women were also warned against pursuing outdoor games. It was not just the threat of the damaging effects of weather on the pale delicate skin of young aristocratic women, or potential accidents and collisions occurring in the game, but the insidious influence of fast running and forceful movement upon their deportment. Lady Greville (1927, p. 18) who, in her regular columns for the *Daily Graphic*, often championed sport as a healthful activity for women, nonetheless considered that

> [g]ames may be excellent for women's health, but they certainly do not make for grace in the drawing-room or for an elegant carriage.

Even those great reformers of female private schooling, Frances Buss at the North London Collegiate School and Miss Beale at Cheltenham Ladies College remained circumspect over advancing competitive outdoor games for their pupils to the same degree as boys. The cultivation of 'grace and elegance of movement' sat alongside educational competence in Miss Buss's goals, dancing being included in the curriculum together with outdoor play, gymnastics, callisthenics and swimming (quoted in McCrone, 1993). Parents needed to be assured that, as well as developing the intellect and health of their daughters, the new provision in education for middle-class females would not exclude them from making a marriage of status. The conservative diet of playing the piano (Solie, 2004), needlework and dancing lessons was perceived to be fundamental to refining a femininity that would appeal to a man in search of a *lady* wife.

The problem for women in the late Victorian ball room

Debutantes' expectations of frequent dances at their first Season balls were often rudely crushed. Uncomfortable in the presence of the opposite sex, and poorly educated in comparison, they might well be passed over for the more socially assured young married women, or the better educated and confident American heiresses in search of a title.[4] Even the spirited Lady Diana Manners, an excellent dancer and a popular partner, had to endure the pains of being ignored (Cooper, 1958, p. 84) in the early days of 'coming out':

> We poor creatures suffered great humiliation, for between dances we joined a sort of slave or marriage market at the door, and those unfortunates with few friends or those who had been betrayed by a partner, or were victims of muddling the sequences of their dances, became cruelly conspicuous wall-flowers.

The experience of the young debutante's first Season's balls was clearly at odds with youthful romantic dreams of being swept into a handsome man's arms to be gently and thrillingly steered around the ball room. Trussed up in tight corsets and pointed shoes, the young debutantes usually lacked experience in conversational ease, were continually subject to the critical scrutiny of the older women and, if asked to dance, had to endure the young men's poor efforts at dancing, as the masculine clumsy feet soiled their satin shoes and ripped their long dresses.

In contrast to men, women were all reputed to like dancing, to have a natural inclination to shine at the activity, which, enhanced by continuous tuition in childhood, supposedly equipped them to salvage the poor dancing of their male peers. The social plight of wallflowers might be improved, a correspondent to the *Daily Graphic* argued,[5] if Society hostesses made more effort to secure introductions for the debutantes. But the male respondents in the ensuing press debate were not so sympathetic. 'One does not go [*to balls*] for the purpose of assisting beginners in practising their steps,' one airily asserted.[6] In any case, a fellow defender of men proposed, the idea that dancing was the principal point of balls was far from the reality:

> [W]omen go to balls to exhibit their dresses, or to enlarge the circle of acquaintance from which they may eventually secure desirable husbands.[7]

If only the young women danced better, another countered in a similar debate several years later, then the men might be more encouraged to participate.

> The single fact of knowing the steps of a dance does not make a good dancer. She must be light and able to adapt herself to any partner,

even a bad one, and thereby make him a better one, and anxious to improve.[8]

Not every woman relished being charged to instruct and lead poor dancers in the ball room. One older woman was clearly shocked when, on being invited to be one half of the top couple in a set of Lancers, she was asked by her partner if she knew the dance. On her startled positive response, the new partner rejoined 'Push me through!'[9] A decade later, a similar situation obtained at court balls. The responsibility of steering their partners through the figures again fell to the women; George V 'expected his aristocracy to avoid false steps in the quadrille as well as in other matters' (Balsan, 1953, p. 31). Outside the systematic training in social dancing received by women within the court circle, however, it was true that female competence in the figures of the Quadrille could not always be guaranteed.

Earlier, in Victoria's reign, Scott argued, most well-bred young women had known how to help their partners around the room. Now, he complained, they were no longer intent on acquiring 'that quiet unostentatious grace that should characterise genuine ball-room dancing'[10] but were selfishly more interested in making an exhibition of their own dancing prowess. Furthermore, contrary to Society etiquette which observed a quiet inclination of the head on greeting fellow dancers in the Quadrille, they indulged in theatrical mannerisms, such as curtseying deeply in square dances, when such forms of obeisance should be reserved to acknowledge royalty. The problem of poor dancing by young women in the ball room, Scott railed, lay with ignorant lady teachers who capitalized on the contemporary craze for 'semi-gymnastic exercises and skirt-dancing'.[11] In agreement, long-established lady teacher, F. R. Hickey, also blamed the parents in this 'age of display' for being content to see very young children 'wave about be-ribboned castanets' at dancing school, rather than be taught the rudiments of social dancing.[12]

Young women dancing in the ball room were as rowdy as the men, complained dancing master Edward Lawson, who was

> inclined to think that many of the systems of the modern gymnasiums and their boisterous exercises may account for some of the decay of graceful actions and conduct, being sometimes too rough and ready for refined young ladies.[13]

Scott was scandalized by the seeming female compliance in rowdy dancing, especially in the Lancers. This 'new war dance,' Scott pronounced, may be fit 'for men and Amazons, or may be for 'New Women,' but certainly not fit for ladies!'[14] Ladies 'should set the fashion' with respect to manners in the ball room advised the Countess of Ancaster, clearly of the widespread opinion that genuine ladies might exercise their 'power ... to promote a good style of dancing';[15] but a younger generation was challenging cultural ideals of gendered movement on the dance floor. In 1891, one correspondent berated debutantes for failing to attract partners. Men had previously acted out of chivalry to amuse women by dancing with them, she argued, but female emancipation in education and careers had dispensed with such a social burden:

> Perhaps the girl has rather to thank herself for this state of affairs. She has asserted her personality; she rides bicycles, she shoots, she wears divided skirts, she dispenses with the solicitous fussiness of the prudent chaperone – and all not quite successfully as an incentive to matrimony.[16]

Some men much preferred ladylike ways: 'the more young women try to imitate their brothers, the more will thoughtful men avoid their society',[17] yet another correspondent tendered a more progressive evaluation of the impact of educational reforms on young women. In the past, 'it was necessary for men to dance with them in order that the conversation might not flag'.[18] Now, he concluded, sitting out the Lancers in order to converse with his partner in the conservatory was a far preferable activity to dancing with her.

Most women, however, were reluctant to relinquish their terpsichorean delights. The answer, they were advised, was to dance with one another.[19] Such a strategy obviously ran counter to the heterosexual ideals of Society balls. From the 1880s, however, opportunities to meet the opposite sex had escalated, far away from the ever-watchful eyes of chaperones and from the strict etiquette of the ball room. For the upper bourgeoisie and the ever-expanding Society, liaisons might now be formed in the more relaxed atmosphere of the numerous sports clubs, most notably lawn tennis, or, even more freely, while bicycling. Young women were now undertaking a far greater range of physical activities, as well as belonging to a wealth of other special interest clubs through which they might pursue art, music, amateur operatics (Lowerson, 2005), and amateur theatricals. But if alternative recreational activities were increasingly available to young wealthy women, their interest in dancing did not necessarily diminish. Opportunities to dance with men at private balls may have become fewer, but young women's love of and association with dancing prevailed. Indeed, 'the girl of the period' the *Pall Mall Gazette* reported in 1892 had grown so independent that, in addition to pursuing sports, she had decided to wait no longer for a dancing man to appear at balls but 'to do without him'.[20] Scott's complaint that young women spent more time learning fancy rather than social dancing was increasingly a point well made.

10
Modelling the Lady

the remarkable *penchant* for fancy dancing.

Dancing, 8 June 1891, p. 1

By the early 1890s fancy dancing was 'regarded as an indispensable adjunct to the list of accomplishments of many of the "upper ten" especially among the fairer sex'.[1] Often requiring the graceful manipulation of a fan, tambourine, scarf or shawl, many fancy dances were designed to develop controlled rounded trajectories of her arms through space (Scott, 1892) and to draw onlookers' attention to her face and figure. At the numerous 'at homes', dinners, garden parties, balls, and charity events, predominantly patronized by Society women, aristocratic and upper-class girls performed the traditional and latest fashionable dances drawn from the professional stage. High-ranking mothers, aunts, and sisters gathered at the public, though still exclusive, charity events such as the regularly reported Children's Salon, launched in 1891 by the editor of *The Gentlewoman*. Each year, the artistic achievements of the 'children of the rich who work for the children of the poor' were judged by well-known professionals.[2] High-class dancing teachers also held 'at homes' in large public venues such as the Queens Gate Hall and Steinway Hall, attracting wide publicity in the Society press and in the specialist women's columns of national newspapers. Performances of their well-heeled young pupils were often individually commented upon, raising the profiles of debutantes, prospective and actual, and eliciting the almost ubiquitous compliments of 'graceful' and 'charming.'

The most fashionable style of fancy dancing during the 1890s was skirt dancing, a genre originated by dancer and choreographer John D'Auban and his sister (Flitch, 1912) during the 1870s. It was, however, the dancing and demeanour of Gaiety Theatre star Kate Vaughan that stimulated a host of imitators both professional and amateur. Replacing the ballet uniform of short, stiff skirts with elegant, ankle-length dresses, under which were several layers of lace petticoats, Vaughan was respected by men and women alike for her elegant and tasteful performances which were held to contrast with the more acrobatic and leg-focused ballet of the period. Her pleasing graceful shapes made by manipulating the fabric in relation to her body revealed no effort. Noted for her tightly corseted slim figure, trademark long black gloves and poetic face, Vaughan exhibited a 'grace that the audiences would wish to see in their own social surroundings and that would serve the ladies of society and the woman of the world' (Michel, 1945, p. 29). Closely aligned with English Society's ideals of ladylike posture, movement, and dress, her performances were much admired by the male aristocracy, one of whom she was later to marry.[3]

Skirt dancing was an ideal vehicle through which to demonstrate ladylike qualities of grace, control, flow, and harmony and, according to one contemporary owed

> half its success to the graceful manipulation of the comparatively long skirt now in vogue, which displays, when judiciously wielded, layers of lace petticoats, which, though ample enough to allow considerable freedom of motion, appear to cling closely to the figure.[4]

It appeared to be a comparatively easy form for amateurs to imitate, for, as one oft-quoted wit declared, the voluminous skirts 'hid a multitude of shins' (see Figure 10.1).

Doctors advised women to take up skirt dancing for their health, while Society columnists emphasized its powers of rejuvenation. Even women over 50, it was rumoured, were taking courses in the form.[5] Dancing teachers and stage dancers advertised lessons, gave demonstrations, choreographed new versions, and published advice on how to dance it. Across the country, young girls rushed to perform in the accordion-pleated skirts made popular by Vaughan's successor Letty Lind in the Gaiety burlesque *Carmen Up to Data*. Skirt dancing had become an indispensable skill for all polite young ladies to perform. Penurious vicar's daughter Winifred Peck (1952, p. 90) dispatched with her sister to be educated at a private young ladies' establishment in Eastbourne, lamented their own late tuition in the art of dancing. In contrast to the more prosperous attendees of the school, drawn from the families of retired army, navy, and business men she realized that they

> were on the wrong side of the gulf which separated the lucky owners of 'accordion-pleated' frocks from those in humdrum outfits.

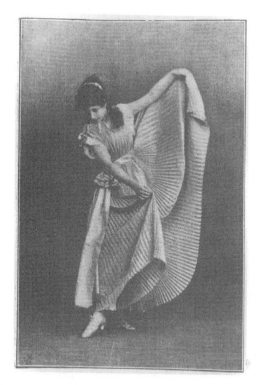

Figure 10.1   Pupil Demonstrating Skirt Dance Position (Scott, *Dancing as an Art and Pastime*, 1892)

> To dance alone in a drawing-room, raising the hem of my skirt to the heavens like a butter-fly, was one of my ambitions never to be fulfilled.

Inspired by the likes of professional skirt dancers Letty Lind, Sylvia Grey, and Topsy Sinden (Flitch, 1912; Hindson, 2007), or themselves former dancers from the musical comedy stage, female teachers schooled their young charges in the basics of fancy dancing and in similar dreams of entering a celebrity stage career. From the mid 1870s, the Gaiety Theatre in its burlesques, operettas, and plays had been influential in advancing before the public a new image of femininity that was respectable and appealing to both Society men and women. Kate Vaughan had been the first of this new breed, deliberately chosen by theatre-owner John Hollingshead to attract Society theatregoers, a strategy continued by his successor George Edwardes. Well-mannered, elegant, beautiful, and always dressed by top London couturiers, Gaiety Girls, though often from comparatively humble origins, were groomed to mix with and, indeed, marry the very best in Society.[6]

Performing before an audience was not, however, restricted to the middle classes, nor was skirt dancing the sole genre taken up by Society. For several centuries, royalty and aristocracy had enjoyed their private theatricals, some even building their own theatres on their country estates or attached to their exclusive London clubs. It was in the magnificent private theatre at the highly exclusive New Club, Covent Garden that aristocratic ladies such as Lady Augusta Fane danced in the late 1880s. Also instrumental in stimulating the 'remarkable penchant for fancy dancing' in Society were the burlesques produced by the Guards at the Royal Theatre, Chelsea Barracks. These featured step dancing, one of the latest fashions in the music halls. Although mostly performed by men, notably the famous comedian and champion step dancer Dan Leno, this percussive, noisy style was also taken up by some Society women, who thereby flew in the face of traditional expectations of ladylike movement.[7]

By the early 1900s, aside from socializing with members of the theatre, titled ladies now danced before the public and debutantes even auditioned to become members of the famous chorus of Gaiety Girls. Changing aristocratic fortunes, personal talent, and ambition, as in the examples of the Countess of Russell and Lady Constance Stewart-Richardson, united in the flow of personnel between the ranks of the aristocracy and the professional theatre. Such socially approved models for young women helped to legitimate the career aspirations of those members of the imitative bourgeoisie who were drawn to the stage and to other arts to pursue a living.[8]

Evoking past gracefulness

Challenges to the social stigma attached to the appearance of women on stage were certainly well in train by the 1890s (Davis, 1991). The conservative values of Mrs Wordsworth's generation and of the court as to what constituted appropriate behaviour and movement for a lady, however, continued to be entertained in many a middle-class drawing room. Models of natural grace for Society women, Mrs Wordsworth (in Grove, 1895, p. 385) exclaimed, voicing the sentiments of many intellectuals, artists, and the class she served, were not to be found in the contemporary era of 'short skirts and acrobatic wonders!'

The ballet of late Victorian Britain (Carter, 2005a) was condemned as having departed from its erstwhile reflection of aristocratic ideals in dress and movement, becoming, in the company of popular entertainment in the music hall, vulgar, artificial, and ugly. Critics considered that too much emphasis was placed on the exposure of the legs, on showy virtuosity, dancing on tip toe and high kicks, rather than the flowing grace and modesty evinced in the dancing of Taglioni and her peers. In spite of loosening public propriety among certain aristocratic and artistic sets in the gay nineties, ballet as a form of exhibition dancing remained beyond the pale for most late Victorian Society women. Ballet girls were reputed to entertain loose morals and engage in prostitution (see Foulkes, 1997), although much of the latter was actually solicited in front of the stage in the promenades of the Alhambra and Empire theatres rather than behind or on its stages. The popular image of the ballet as a profession that ranked with the oldest was slow to vanish. The late Victorian ballet uniform of short and often transparent skirts that revealed the legs up to and above the knee was considered indecent and vulgar by Society; though the nakedness of the limbs was suggestive rather than actual, given that the dancers wore flesh-coloured tights. Small wonder that Mrs Wordsworth was adamant that the refined training in dancing that she gave to her Society pupils was most emphatically not a preparation for a stage career. Instead, she advocated a return to Hellenic principles.

The dancing of the ancient Greeks, even though no easily workable primary records existed, was an inspirational and important factor in the late Victorian and Edwardian pursuit of artistic, healthy and beautiful dancing. Growing appreciation of naturalness in movement, much of which drew from a Romantic equation of beauty, honesty and gracefulness with nature, and sentiments popularised by the widely read Herbert Spencer (1950) in his essays on beauty and gracefulness prompted dancers, artists, and teachers to reinvigorate such values for contemporary society. This vein of thought, not peculiar to Britain, but active across European and North American culture, was to find overt expression in the next generation of concert dancing in the figures of Isadora Duncan, Ruby Ginner and Margaret Morris (see, for example, Ruyter, 1979; Fensham and Carter (2011); Macintosh, 2010).

Victorian fascination with classical ideals corresponded with deeply held convictions that European civilization owed its global supremacy to such origins, a view that pervaded respectable society as an education in classics reached greater numbers of the bourgeoisie. Cultivating, through dance and gesture, the natural movement and posture attributed to the ancient Greeks was deemed educational, potentially physically transformative, and morally improving, as well as a pleasurable pastime. 'The postures of these classic times were the perfection of grace', Mrs Wordsworth (in Grove, 1895, p. 385) declared. The statues of Venus de Medici and Hercules were similarly advocated by Scott (1887b) as inspiration for contemporary youth.

Illustrating Mrs Wordsworth's notes on dancing (in Grove, 1895) are photographs of young women, dressed in flowing Greek robes, holding cymbals and rope garlands. In one illustration, captioned 'Graceful Movement, No. 2' (p. 383) the young dancer poses for the camera, front foot pointed, upper back arched, in her raised hand a cymbal, her arm framing her face as she gazes out to the reader. The image is reminiscent of earlier Victorian photography and of the popular fashion for *tableaux vivants* in which scenes of antiquity and of venerated paintings of the old masters (themselves inspired by Greek art and mythology) presented women in decorative, but culturally approved, attitudes. Through the discriminating study of all forms of dancing, past and present, Mrs Wordsworth hoped that 'a new golden age of dancing may open out for England, when instead of comparing a dancer to a Greek statue, one may see in the perfect pose and movement a new type of English beauty' (in Grove, 1895, p. 386). Implicit in Mrs Wordsworth's text and its illustrations is an unquestioned acceptance that dancing, moral health, and beauty are intrinsically female. If contemporary English society aimed to progress away from degeneration towards a renewal of civilization, then appropriate schooling of high-class young ladies in the manners and stately dances of a more courtly society might lead, through example, to a wider renewal in good taste, decorum and beauty.

A more demonstrable civilized past lay in the eighteenth century. Classical ideals of grace, harmony, and proportion, as social and moral qualities as well as aesthetic, were thought to be consequent with the dancing of the eighteenth-century ball room. The paradox here was, of course, that French deportment had been castigated as too artificial and consequently insincere by advocates of English honest simplicity in etiquette and business affairs – but the distance of years lent a softly hued focus to pre-industrial times and even to the manners of the despotic court of England's old enemy. For Scott, the person of Marie Antoinette, viewed as the last of her female kind in a more polite and cultured world, served as an ideal of unaffected, natural though sophisticated deportment for young women, rather than as an autocratic and morally indulgent relic of the ancient regime.

Royal tutor Louis D'Egville considered instruction in old ceremonial dances such as the Minuet, Gavotte, and Pavane to be 'effective both on the stage and in the drawing-room, and ... moreover, extremely useful in the class-room as a means of teaching balance and quiet grace'

(D'Egville in Grove, 1895, p. 422). The *pièce de resistance* among historical dances was the Menuet de la Cour, a late eighteenth-century legacy,
still in the repertoire of several Society dancing teachers (Russell and
Bourassa, 2007). Initially choreographed as a stage dance, it was adopted
by the French court in the 1770s to exhibit studied refinement and grace
in dancing. During the 1830s and 1840s, the Menuet de la Cour, often
coupled with its near contemporary the Gavotte de Vestris (Hammond,
1984), returned to the theatre as a showpiece for famous ballerinas Fanny
Elssler, Lucile Grahn (both usually performing *en travesti*), Fanny Cerrito,
and, less frequently, Marie Taglioni. Years later, Margaret Rolfe described
the much hyped and long awaited 'real' Menuet de la Cour as executed
by her teacher as exceptionally slow and boring. By the 1890s, the Menuet
de la Cour enjoyed further currency, often choreographed anew in solo,
couple and Quadrille forms for the stage and salon. Nor was there any
necessity to wear special costumes for the after dinner entertainment.
Rather than singing, women now danced for fellow guests in their fashionable evening gowns, for as Elizabeth Garratt observed: 'a dress with
a train does beautifully for a minuet'.[9]

As oral memories and kinetic tradition of eighteenth-century deportment and dancing faded, languid postures and mincing steps in historical pageants, plays, and dedicated concerts evoked for the late Victorians
a lost civil and decorous age. The irony was that, although summoning
the shades of times when kings and queens danced in social and political rituals, the actual effect was to remove dancing yet further from the
interests of men who wished to wield power. As an aesthetic spectacle,
dancing became the domain of the disempowered: women and children.
It was not an image that might lure the late Victorian man back into the
ball room, for in the image of 'olde worlde' charm he might perceive
neither his reflection nor ambition. It did, however, present before his
eyes a vision of unchallenging prettiness, a harmless, ornamental spectacle at which he might gaze, looking for a potential wife or mistress.
Hitherto, opportunities to stare at women while they danced had been
mainly restricted to the ballet, the music hall, or popular theatre where,
earlier in the century, no woman of good reputation would tread.

11
Where Are Our Men?

> For my own part, I do not like to see a gentleman dance
> *too well*; he does not want to be taken for a dancing-
> master. It is enough if he dance *like a gentleman*.
> The Lounger in Society, *The Glass of Fashion*,
> 1881, p. 164

At the beginning of the nineteenth century, it was generally accepted among Society that the well-bred gentleman appeared as a man of refinement who carried himself with unaffected graceful ease, knew how to dance, and how to interact with women. By the end of Victoria's reign, these ideals of polite masculine behaviour were in disarray among the very social group who had long acted as a model for the rest of society. No single reason is identifiable for this contestation. Decline in the performance of gentlemanly masculinity was a long, complex, and often contradictory process (Tosh, 1999, 2005a, 2005b). Crucially, it was a significant factor in the transformation in the status of dancing in political, economic, and social life. The ideal of male aristocratic carriage and behaviour in the ballroom, however, remained a pervasive influence into the twentieth century, as the cult of gentility was espoused lower down the social scale as a sign of social distinction.

Throughout Victoria's reign, the concept of the gentleman was to be radically re-worked, shifting from the more cosmopolitan eighteenth-century concept of the man of manners to the Victorian man of action, the quintessential English gentleman. But the transition was never smooth, never uniformly observed, or, indeed, within the conservative circles of Society and the middle classes fully accepted. Within more conservative circles, there was often a sense of nostalgia and regret at the loss of what appeared to be the refined male conduct of an earlier, more civilized age, believed to have reached its apotheosis in the previous century.

The true gentleman, the aristocrat, attired in fashionable yet unostentatious dress, was identifiable by his posture and gait, ideally characterized by a quiet elegance and grace. Early in life, he had learned how to distinguish his movement range and energy from that of his female partner, and how to treat her publicly in a chivalrous yet unaffected manner. For those born outside the rank and title of gentleman, the acquisition of this cultural capital from a 'school of dancing and good manners' (Henderson [1879], p. ix) was considered to help the aspiring gentleman to move with ease in Society, affording him greater confidence in quotidian interactions and increasing his potential to attract a wife of higher social status. Moving *like* a gentleman, even when not born into such a privileged class, held out prospects of acceptance *as* a gentleman.

Moving like a gentleman

Views on men and dancing, such as those from the seventeenth century philosopher John Locke and eighteenth-century dance theorist John Weaver, were quoted wholesale or paraphrased without acknowledgement in numerous dancing manuals, books on etiquette, and instructional literature. Frequently cited was the Earl of Chesterfield's (1783) instruction:

> Next to good breeding is genteel manners and carriage and the best method to acquire these is through knowledge of dance. Now to acquire a graceful air, you must attend to your dancing; no one can sit, stand or walk well, unless you dance well. And in learning to dance, be particularly attentive to the motion of your arms for stiffness in the wrist will make any man look awkward. If a man walks well, presents himself well in company, wears his hat well, moves his head properly, and his arms gracefully, it is almost all that is necessary.[1]

Such advice was recycled in a literature market designed for the rising middle classes. That close association between correct dancing and deportment as a ticket to circulation in polite society echoed across the nineteenth century. In 1861, for example, Mme D'Egville Michau (p. 33) advocated that every

> boy should learn dancing, as it gives him an ease of manner he seldom attains without ... They must learn to enter and leave a room

properly, hand a lady through a dance with ease, and take off their hats like gentlemen. Do these simple acts naturally and gracefully, and they will also look like gentlemen.

Prescriptive manuals concurred that above all, the gentleman should not call attention to himself on the dance floor, either by adopting an affected manner or by executing large or rushed movements. Sudden or jerky actions were not at all desirable; even the necessarily more energetic steps of elevation were to be performed in a restrained manner fairly close to the floor, so that the elegant demeanour of the dancer was not disturbed. Gentlemen should stand upright, the head centred and erect, the arms held straight by the sides of the body in a relaxed manner, and, as Crompton ([1891], p. 32) recommended, the elbows were never to be bent 'outward, so as to create awkward and unseemly angles, which are as displeasing to the eye as they are destitute of grace.' Both on and off the dance floor, the gentleman must walk confidently and smoothly, using a larger stride than that of a woman, his knees neither locked stiffly, nor worse still, bent and bandy-legged. His legs were to be turned outwards, moving easily from the hip, the toes pointing downwards, and his knees, when purposefully bent, should be kept in line with the toes. Such technical stipulations were fully in accord with the fundamentals of ballet technique. Once in the ball room, on inviting a lady onto the floor, a gentleman was expected to present his hand with the palm uppermost, and then, when in Waltz positions, support his partner with his arm encircling her upper back, while always avoiding close bodily contact. Deviation from such rules suggested a man who ran the social stigma of failing either to *be* or *act like* a gentleman.

There had long been a tension between the ideal and the reality of gentility: though the well-bred were considered to be born elegant and graceful, they nonetheless needed to learn specific aristocratic movement codes, using the services of someone below their social station, to fashion their bodily superiority. Natural ease actually needed the hard work of art. This aesthetic harked back to the ideals of the French aristocratic court where political and aesthetic ideologies (Cohen, 2005; McGowan, 2008) dictated that the manifestation of true gentility resided in art successfully masquerading as nature. The illogicality of using art to appear as if naturally fashioned was circumnavigated in the discourse of dancing teachers by suggesting that the inherent aptitude of the well-bred required a little polishing, preferably from an early age.

Mrs Henderson's ([1879], p. vi) twentieth edition of her ball room guide asserts that

> [n]ature alone will not teach good manners. Art is nature's younger sister, and comes in to finish what Nature begins ... With Nature alone we are awkward and simple – with Art alone we are formal, cold and deceitful.

In cultivating this pretence of grace as the outward bodily manifestation of noble birth, there was a continuing insistence upon minimal effort being displayed:

> [e]ase of manner, perfectly free from constraint, but entirely removed from either affectation or effrontery, is an essential requisite in a gentleman.[2]

'[T]here must be no evidence that the movement or posture is a matter of consideration to the person making it, or all the effect will be destroyed' determined Scott (1887a, pp. 35–6). The manifestation of effort, energetic and large, unrestrained movements suggested the lower orders of society who, the upper and middle classes believed, were naturally coarse and vulgar in their movement.

Grace could though, Scott admitted, result from 'constant practice' rather than a natural accomplishment (1887a, p. 35), but the majority of etiquette guides cautioned against the visibility of practice: the genuine gentleman should be wary of demonstrating too much polish in his movements. Visible energy expenditure and large movements could betray an acquired rather than innate facility, indicative of an artificially constructed persona, a man aiming to pass as a *gentle*man, but whose studied movements did not arise from the reality or sincerity of his position. Following the French and Industrial Revolutions, the paradox of artificial training to render a body natural was not lost on a nation that valued honesty in all aspects of life, and that became increasingly suspicious of elaborate movement codes in social interaction, regarding them as a device to disguise true intention. Such devious strategies of bodily subterfuge were not reckoned by the English bourgeoisie, in particular, to be typical of the English gentleman, but, in xenophobic fashion, were regarded as peculiar to the foreigner, especially the French.[3]

In addition to being taken for a foreigner, a man who paid attention to extremes of neatness and detail in his dancing might run the risk of being identified as a working artist, not a leisured gentleman.[4] That social aesthetic is perhaps best captured in Byron's oft-quoted description of his hero's dancing prowess in *Don Juan* published in 1823:

> He danced without theatrical pretence,
> Not like a ballet-master in the van
> Of his drill'd nymphs, but like a gentleman.
>
> *Don Juan* (canto XIV, stanza 38)

At the end of the century, Edward Scott (1892, p. 133) recounted a new pupil's misgivings about earlier tuition. The pupil confessed:

> "I do not doubt that Mister —— understands dancing and teaching dancing well enough; but somehow I am under the impression that he is not accustomed to teaching *gentlemen*".

Scott noted in the pupil's demonstration 'a general air of affectation and staginess, a style that would have appeared altogether out of place in a drawing-room' and triumphantly commended the 'innate sense of refinement' that led him, unlike his friend, to seek out instruction from a dancing master experienced in teaching 'strictly in accordance with the principles of good taste'.

But if aping the style of theatrical dancers was to be studiously avoided, so too was closely following the model of the dancing master himself, for fear of being taken for the teacher rather than the pupil. To avoid similar misidentification, young men in Society during the 1870s were warned neither to appear too familiar with cotillion figures, nor to attend numerous or late night cotillion parties on the edges of their cultural circle (Boyle, 1873). If, however, the young gentleman failed to be successful in these dance party games, he might court ridicule from people outside his class, and appear particularly foolish in front of women. Anxiety over the potential shame caused by failure and incompetence on the dance floor was recurrently voiced by men in the closing decades of the nineteenth century. Taken with other developments in male socialization and gender relations in the period, it is clear that, despite the greater volume of publishing outlets for the expression of opinion, new concerns were being added to long-standing worries over being mistaken as a member of the lower classes, as a theatrical dancer, or as a dancing master.

The problem with men in the ball room

Nineteenth-century etiquette stipulated that men should do more than merely dance at a ball; they should participate fully in looking after the pleasures of others. As Society commentator Mrs Humphry (1897a, p. 103) opined:

> [t]he delight of the average hostess's heart is the well-bred man, unspoiled by conceit, who can always be depended on to do his duty.

In return for the hospitality of a free supper and champagne, men were expected to arrive in good time, introduce themselves to the hostess, take up her suggestions for partners, dance with the daughter of the house, and above all, promise to dance with those women they had agreed to partner at the appointed moment. They were further required to make light conversation and return their partner to her seat at a dance's conclusion or take her for refreshments, if she so wished. When supper was announced, they were obliged to accompany their dance partner to the table and look after her needs; or provide an apology and a substitute if they had contracted a previous engagement to conduct someone else to supper. Above all, young men were instructed to spread themselves evenly and unselfishly among the female guests as gallant dance partners and escorts.

In the century's closing decades, this code of the Society ball room was often breached (see, for example, Boyle, 1873). In the press and reminiscences of the period, grievances against young men recur: they arrived late and ignored the young eligible women; they preferred to talk among themselves or to older women; they rarely danced and if they did, it was poorly; they hung around *en masse* and avoided introductions; they failed to look after the needs of their partners; they remained seated, while the ladies stood; they spent too much time and consumed too much food and drink at the supper table; and to cap it all, they left immediately after supper without returning to partner the young ladies in the ball room.

References abound to the 'black phalanx' of men in evening dress who cluttered up doorways, lounged around the edges of the room, or sat on the staircase, failed to ask the women to dance, and whose attitude was described as bored, vacant looking, rude, snobbish, and ill-mannered. Such a state of affairs provoked considerable discussion in an effort to identify the causes of such behaviour and to find urgent remedies to repair the social contract. Young men were integral to the success of the

London Season but, as the matriarchs of the Upper Ten fretted, their refusal to dance placed the continuity of Society in jeopardy.

Scholars examining the historical trajectory of dance and gender in Eurocentric society have tended to focus upon theatrical and concert dance contexts (Burt, 2007; Banes, 1998) where ideological issues of gender construction and the male gaze have often been favoured in the exposition. By examining social contexts for dancing, it becomes possible to expand existing analyses of dance and masculinity and gain a more nuanced and fulsome understanding, not only of ideological but also material contributory factors. As historian Richard Holt (2006) has trenchantly observed with respect to studies of the parallel growth of amateur sports in Britain, too little attention has been paid to concomitant material and environmental conditions. In a society undergoing rapid industrialization and urbanization, there were unprecedented shifts in the use of time and space that impacted on human bodies across all classes of society, although obviously not in a uniform manner. Society young men at the end of the nineteenth century were by no means unaffected by such developments and their perceptions and experiences of the physical demands and constraints in the ball room need to be examined as part of the often contradictory complex of factors that both reflected and was constitutive of male attitudes towards dancing.

The immediate physical environment of the ballroom was often cited as a reason for not dancing. Society young men protested against charges of laziness, complaining that the rooms were often too crowded and too hot for dancing (Williams, 1892). Such excuses were by no means ill founded. Society's relaxation of its own boundaries and the desire of new hostesses to demonstrate their social position and popularity frequently resulted in overcrowding. Advised in the Society press and in etiquette books to invite more men than women to ensure a plentiful supply of partners, hostesses packed guests into domestic drawing rooms that had not been designed for the physical activity of large groups of people. The small windows were often closed, even in the summer months, for fear that those seated or over exerting themselves might catch a chill from the draught.

Nor was the men's attire conducive to energetic dancing. The starched high collars, neckties, pointed dancing shoes, long-tailed black evening coat, and white gloves constituted a uniform, any element of which a man could not remove in public, regardless of circumstance; it hardly bore comparison with the new sports clothes that were designed for ease of movement and comfort. Men's evening dress, likened to a straitjacket by one dancing man, changed little over the decades.[5] Indeed, it was rendered even more uncomfortable during the 1890s with the brief return in fashion to corsets for men.

In the voluminous debate, tiredness was frequently cited by the young men for their failure to participate. Characteristically, Scott (1892, p. 124) dismissed such protestations as 'laziness, sheer laziness that is at the bottom of it'. But several commentators took these concerns at face value and worried about the apparent declining physical health of young men. Contrasting the contemporary lack of vigour in the ball room with the energy displayed by earlier generations, one discussant pointed to the changing demands since the previous century made upon aristocratic men in terms of physical fitness in their daily lives. Formerly, he argued, young aristocratic men retained levels of fitness through managing their country estates outdoors. Such nostalgic comparisons were given short shrift by others who countered accusations of physical decline by pointing to young men's physical activities on the sports field.[6]

Other commentators worried that the failure to dance among 'indolent youth' was evidence of a deep-seated moral and physical malaise that was symptomatic of degeneration. Yet others argued that this tiredness reflected disaffection with the unvarying ball room repertoire. When young people began to enliven the procedures through the energetic style that opponents termed 'rowdyism', however, their performance only brought fresh censure from critics who grumbled about declining standards. Whether absenting themselves entirely from the dance floor or throwing themselves with gusto into the established dances of the day, young men were judged to be reneging in their social competence and duty.

In some cases though, these complaints of tiredness were indeed more than affectation and reflected a genuine disquiet, particularly among those now employed by the City, at the lateness of the hours regularly adopted at London balls. Getting up early to travel to the office was not helped by going to bed at dawn. Furthermore, who one had danced with the night before might add to the man's feelings of exhaustion. Most young men preferred to dance with a slim, pretty girl who could dance well, but inevitably, this ideal was not available to all. Society compunction to treat all women fairly required men to dance with large women, whether tall or corpulent, who might require considerable effort to steer around the floor. *Punch's* cartoons often depicted this gap between the ideal and the reality, illustrating a young man's predicament or avoidance strategy when presented with a large, middle-aged partner, who was far from the belle of the ball.[7]

Physical size, nonetheless, was not always indicative of the likely dancing experience. How the woman positioned herself and moved within

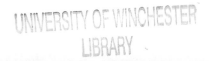

her partner's arms might often belie her actual size and weight. The most portly of matrons might prove to be as light as a feather on the dance floor while, after partnering the slenderest of damsels, a man might feel that he had just heaved a sack of potatoes around the room. 'What's her dancing weight?' anxiously enquires one dancing man on a hot afternoon, 'this isn't the weather for fourteen stone'.[8] Certain women proved a real trial to navigate around the ballroom: leaning on the gentleman's shoulder, nipping his arm with their left elbow, or pulling away from him too forcefully at the waist (Scott, 1887a). These examples of poor technique frequently caused the men to nurse an aching arm the morning after the ball. Such discomfort, coupled with the late hours, drove many knights of the ball room to pronounce dancing to be literally not worth the candle.

This all presupposed that the men actually possessed the competence to dance, or at least the inclination to take regular lessons from a reputable teacher. One dissatisfied young woman observed that there were to be found ten types of dancing man at a ball: 'one who can dance, and nine who can't. The one who can is generally to be found in the supper-room'.[9] Very often, the men eschewed taking lessons: 'too much of a bore' and 'too much trouble'.[10] Certainly, learning how to dance properly necessitated an outlay in time and money in which a growing number of men were reluctant to invest. Instead, they often muddled around the dance floor, basing their knowledge on limited observation of more competent male dancers, the favours of sisters or friends to provide impromptu lessons, or else the patience and goodwill of experienced female partners to guide them through the figures of the Quadrille. *Punch's* artists capitalized on female society's disaffection with recalcitrant male dancers: in one cartoon, the young blood enthuses to his partner how frequently he dances at Society events: 'I wonder you don't learn!' is his exasperated companion's barbed response.[11]

Dancing teachers, angered by declining standards and dwindling demands for their services, accused the men of meanness, complaining that in those instances where expert help was sought, the young men turned to the cheapest bidder, expecting that one quick course was sufficient for life. The trade in teaching dances rather than the art of dancing remained Scott's bugbear throughout his long career; yet male dancers frequently sought the quick, cheap alternative, one prospective pupil, indeed, requesting only to be taught those dances 'in which he holds the girl round the waist!'[12] Faced with so many complaints from women about their lack of dancing prowess, some men retaliated that the fault lay with the women, not with them. Too many young women, complained one man, relied too much upon what they had learned at dancing school and were unable to deviate from it. Men in contrast, he argued, preferred to follow their own lead and expected the women to follow.[13] But to cut a figure on the dance floor required aptitude, lessons, practice, and, increasingly, a willingness to stand out from the crowd. For the typical young men of late Victorian Society, in spite of frequent entreaties and laments from female dancers and hostesses, there was comparatively little in the ball room to induce the 'lords of creation' to make the effort.

12
Dancing Dogs and Manly Men

> I like to see decision and vigour exhibited in a man's
> dancing, an air of confidence and repose, as if he had
> thorough control over his movements.
>
> Scott, *Grace and Folly*, 1887b, p. 121

The late Victorian exodus of men from the fashionable ball room was
by no means absolute; a significant number of men continued to love
dancing. Viscount Esher (1927) recounts in his memoirs how he and a
fellow undergraduate regularly caught the early morning train back to
Cambridge after an extravagant ball at some great house in the capital;
George Cornwallis West, second husband of Lady Churchill, was remem-
bered as the best dancer in London and Princess Alexandra herself enjoyed
the partnership of several courtiers. Oliver Montagu, equerry to the Prince
of Wales, was reputedly a wonderful role model for young men aspiring
to behave impeccably as knights of old in the ball room, epitomizing the
romantic ideal that 'nothing makes a girl look so well in a ball-room as
a good partner'.[1] Yet an increasing number of young Society men were
turning their backs on the dance floor.

The dancing man to the rescue

Society hostesses became desperate to secure partners for their female
guests, proffering invitations to young men who were known dancers, but who in previous decades would not have been eligible to rub
shoulders with select company. Dancing skill enabled a well-turned out
young man with contacts to enter Society events where he might avail
himself of the opportunity to share free entertainment, a chance to meet
young girls, and to consume a free supper. A new breed was identified

by Society and its press: the dancing man. His terpsichorean abilities were not, however, his only distinguishable feature: the dancing man's appearance and conduct also marked him as a distinct species. Male evening dress with its long-tailed black coat and trousers, black or white waistcoat, white shirt, and gloves had become *de rigueur* by this period for all formal dance occasions, but even within the confines of this uniform, the dancing man was easily distinguishable. Subject of a number of satirical sketches in *Punch* and other press, he was typically depicted in fashionable evening wear, with a tightened waist, waxed moustache and neatly styled hair, a very high white starched collar, tight trousers, and pointed dancing pumps. But the added detail of solitaire diamonds worn at the breast and impeccably clean gloves, to which the wearer paid much attention, singled out the dancing man.[2]

So too did his conduct, though complaints against the 'dancing dogs' tended to arise from his male peers rather than from the women.[3] The dancing man was depicted as vain, supercilious, and essentially selfish in seeking to enjoy himself, rather than to afford pleasure to others, regardless of their terpsichorean prowess. Having studied the 'style, steps, and capabilities of the various ladies, he makes his selections, and reserves his favours for those alone' displaying no interest in his partners or in conversation beyond dancing.[4] Some critics of the 'dancing man' considered him guilty of actually causing the crisis in the ball room by placing too great a premium on the technical demands of dancing. By the end of the 1890s, however, even this phenomenon of the rarefied type of dancing man was becoming scarce in Society ball rooms, if contemporary cartoons can be believed.[5]

Ultimately, the problem with men in the ball room did not lie inside its walls but outside. It was not competence in dancing alone that held them back from the dance floor, but, above all, changing gender relations and new leisure opportunities that rendered the Society ball room an artificial and constrained space in which to spend and express their youth. Throughout the nineteenth century, the social and cultural construction of aristocratic and upper-bourgeois masculinity had been slowly moving away from the realm of the family and the private tutor towards the public institutions of exclusively male schools and clubs where distinctive modes of play became key in socializing the aristocratic and entrepreneurial men of the British Empire.

New trends in socializing the male upper classes

The history of aristocratic education in the nineteenth century is remarkable for the systematic development of the public school (Honey, 1977).

These private boarding establishments existed in the previous century, but it was not until the mid-Victorian period that it became increasingly common among the upper classes to send their boys away to school. Specific preparation for the public school was undertaken by private tuition, often by sons of clergymen. Dancing was not offered at the most elite of the public schools, Eton College, Harrow School, and Winchester College – and indeed in the early nineteenth century, the curriculum at each varied in provision overall.[6] Emphasis was, however, on the mental rather than physical education of the boy, long hours being spent learning by rote in the school room.

Inspired by the reforms of Matthew Arnold at Rugby School, by the 1850s a system of curriculum, discipline, and values came to be shared among the nine public schools that were regarded as the best of the nation. The public school sector is particularly notable for its development of organized games, displacing the earlier, somewhat free and anarchic leisure time enjoyed by the boys, and training in the gentlemanly arts of fencing and boxing. The inclusion of organized sports appears to have been born of the enthusiasm of the particular masters appointed at schools such as Uppingham and Rugby, although earlier it was introduced largely as a means of cultivating discipline among the unruly boys. The inclusion of organized sports was initially an elite form of rational recreation and only later did the rationale of manliness and male bonding in preparation for adult life emerge. This was to lead to the cult of athleticism in the public school (Mangan, 2008), driving a further nail into the coffin of male aristocratic education in dance.

Over the century, a system reflecting these values came into being: the preparatory school, public school, and university. Not all public schoolboys were automatically expected to go on to university; aristocrats acquired places at Eton and Harrow and later at Oxford and Cambridge as a birthright. They then moved into positions of governance. It was a system of which the newly rising merchant classes were envious. If the fathers had not enjoyed such privileges in their own schooling, then they were determined that their sons would follow such a pathway (Wiener, 1981). Through the education system of privilege, the sons of aristocrats, gentry, and the comparatively few well-to-do upper-middle class established a network, distinctive accent and shared memories and traditions that would assist them in their social world.

Young aristocratic boys were instructed in dance at home alongside their sisters before attending preparatory school, though some continued to be educated completely by home tutors until late in the nineteenth century. Dancing classes, both compulsory and optional, had

appeared on the curriculum of many eighteenth-century schools that
catered principally for the boys of gentry and the emerging mercan-
tile classes (Caffyn, 1998; Leppert, 1988). Over the next century, these
increasingly contracted from a full academic year to a term, schools preferring to offer games, gymnastics, and even drill throughout the year
as a means of promoting physical health and education. In the autumn
term, dancing teachers struggled to equip the boys with sufficient dancing skills for the round of parties during the Christmas holidays, but the
10 or 12 classes amounting to around fifteen hours at most were clearly
inadequate.[7] Competing with other festive entertainment, supplemen-
tary Christmas holiday classes often failed to engage the boys' regular
attendance and concentration.

There were, however, ideological reasons that caused an aversion to
dancing classes that were rooted in the constructions of masculinity and
femininity enshrined in the Victorian education system and curriculum. Public school boys were prepared for a future life in public service,
whether running the country, their own estates, the church, or the military. The educational system fostered a particular form of male bonding
that equipped the boys with shared experiences and values as the future
ruling class, but simultaneously devalued their former lives within the
bosom of the family. Excluded from the new world of the public school
were mothers, nurses, governesses, sisters, and brothers yet too young to
attend; females and children who ranked low in the power stakes. As a
consequence, activities enjoyed by these latter groups declined in their
cultural *cachet*.

Exclusively male in their membership and located in their own permanent premises, London clubs in the late nineteenth century proved an
important development in upper- and middle-class male social intercourse
(Taddei, 1999). Spacious and comfortable, the clubs were principally positioned in the St James area, near to Society's hub, close to government, and
to one another so that gentlemen might enjoy the benefits of membership of more than one. They provided a focal meeting place for men of
like minds or similar experiences, each club professing a central interest
as political, military, sporting, artistic, literary, university, public school,
occupational, or social. The latter were the most select, since they required
no other eligibility test than that of status or connection. Entry to all clubs
was by a set fee and annual subscription, the cost of which, to a limited
extent, restricted access. In the main, however, social exclusivity was largely
controlled by election (see Figure 12.1).

Membership was greatly coveted by the rising middle class. Between
1860 and 1900 membership of London clubs increased in a parallel

132

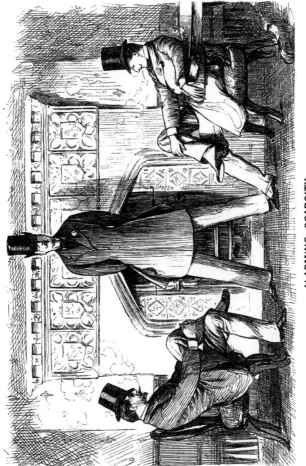

ALARMING SCARCITY.

Scene—*Club Smoking-Room.*

First Young Swell. " Aw !—going anywhere ? "

Second Ditto. " No !—asked to ten ' Hops' to-night ! The Idea has completely floored me ! "

Third Ditto. " By Jove ! I've been thinking of letting myself out at Ten Pounds a Night. A fellow might recoup himself for a bad Book on the Derby."

Figure 12.1 Alarming Scarcity, *Punch*, 11 July 1874

development with the expansion of Society. As Britain emerged into full economic and imperial power, businessmen of large and, indeed, those of lesser fortune sought equivalent social status and influence to the aristocracy through the opportunities afforded by the club. Membership conferred a sense of equality and acceptance so that access to aristocrats, politicians, lawyers, bankers, and merchants on an individual basis was more easily accomplished than through the system of introductions at Society events. The club served a similar social function to that of Society. It proved 'a ready-made means for social intercourse, an information network, and a source of societal status' (Taddei, 1999, p. 15). It also provided a sanctuary away from feminine control and feminine custom. Given the late Victorian tendency to delay marriage until well into the twenties, young men, without wife and house, were dependent on the amenities of the club. Providing premises, catering, and accommodation, this all-male environment released the bachelor from obligation to Society hostesses. No longer did they need to attend balls for a good supper in exchange for partnering female guests.[8] At the club, young men could enjoy their pleasures without female censure, many then going on to seek late night clubs of dubious repute at which freer styles of dancing might figure and more open associations with women, smoking, drinking, and gambling be pursued.

But if Society men did take to the floor, it was becoming a trend to dance badly as a badge of honour: 'caun't dawnce, dammit' was the fashionable drawl of Society youth, regardless of opportunity. During the late 1870s, as man-about-town Ralph Nevill (1912) recalled, a distinct set among fashionable youth assumed boredom and lack of effort in all activities. This pronounced imitation of the leisured life of the aristocrat was stereotypical of the dandy, the aesthete, who emerged as an embodied critique of bourgeois and conventional life (Moers, 1960; Adams, 1995). As dancing became an increasing leisure pursuit for the middle classes, too much enthusiasm for its practice at Society balls might suggest compliance with convention, pointing towards the very bourgeois cult of rule-bound gentility. More prosaically, some fashion-conscious young men were loathe to ruffle their appearance by dancing at Society balls. A correspondent to *The Daily Graphic* in 1891 queried whether it was conceivable that

> any sane tailor-and-hosier-made young man would imperil his immaculate shirt-front and collar by joining the scramble in the middle of a West-end ballroom.[9]

Movement codes for the male aristocracy were by no means homogeneous. Over and above family and personalized inflections of moving were distinctly masculine bodies and movement systems that were designed for life outside of the court and Society ball rooms. Chief of these were the sports field and the military, domains in which considerable numbers of male aristocracy were active. *Punch*, for example, satirized the inappropriate transference of energies and movement trajectories from the rugby pitch to the ball room, as well as the language and expectations of the military drill master employed to train school girls in physical culture.[10] In spite of the frequency of military balls, providing ample opportunity for practice, the military man was not by the end of the century regarded as an able dancer. Famously, the Prince of Wales's own regiment, the Tenth Hussars, was known as the 'Don't Dance Tenth'. The figure of the military man on the dance floor became one that lent itself to satire rather than admiration. Daily training in military drill and the inclusion of athletics and gymnastics in the military programme did not equip a man to move easily around the nineteenth-century ball room. His over-erect and stiff bearing, bound movement, and lack of experience in moving in close proximity to another person, whom he then had to steer, were antithetical to cutting a fine figure on the dance floor.[11]

If a gentleman were to take to the dance floor, it was crucial for his good standing that on no account should he draw undue attention to himself. Male reluctance to employ more than a modicum of energy on the dance floor chimed with long-standing recommendations against being taken for a professional or member of the lower class. Singer Hayden Coffin recalled the ideal dancer of the 1880s as one who 'could go round the room with a glass of water on his head and not spill a drop'.[12]

This feature of dancing with the aim of 'not leaving a hair unturned at the end' was considered a specifically English trait by a Belgian observer resident in London in the 1890s. Her evaluation, while suggesting that the English prefer not to expend energy unduly without obvious reward, also pointed to the fear of self-exhibitionism. Contrasting the energy and frequent vocalizations of enjoyment of Scotsmen dancing, she believed Englishmen to be 'afraid of attracting attention, and being laughed at'.[13] This anxiety is captured in the no doubt apocryphal observation that 'an Englishman never dances alone unless he is intoxicated, and then he is taken into custody'.[14] As an Englishman, dancing was strictly an activity to be undertaken with a female partner. 'We dance strictly to please young girls' opined a columnist calling himself John Bull in *Punch* earlier in the century, noting that the 'more grave is any man's profession, the more dignified his office, the more odd and strange is the idea of that man dancing'.[15] Men holding dignified office, though, were expected to dance at ceremonial events such as state balls during the Victorian period, though solo performances were thought best left to theatricals. '[A]nything savouring of the theatre, of artistic form, is tabooed' lamented dancing master Edward Humphrey of young men in 1902.[16]

Undoubtedly the homosociality that was encouraged in the public school system contributed to this fear of appearing foolish in public. Crompton pointed to the absence of compulsory dancing lessons at Eton and Harrow which rendered young men incompetent in the ballroom. On leaving school, Crompton argued, the young man is reluctant 'to play once more the boy' by taking lessons, and on seeing the 'awkward figure some of his friends cut ... vows that *he* is not going to make a fool of himself, and ever after "dancing is too much trouble for him"'.[17] Such anxiety was not only attributable to peer pressure; men were particularly apprehensive that they would be laughed at by women. Such sensitivities are perhaps understandable given the courtship role accorded to dancing at Society functions, but this fear of attracting female ridicule was manifest much earlier in life. As one Society mother commented of boys attending dancing classes in the 1890s: 'they look so foolish wobbling about before the young lady teaching them'.[18] For the future rulers of Empire, such loss of face in front of those who were positioned lower in the power stakes produced no incentive to learn.

In any case, the young men were more proficient at and found greater enjoyment in their team sports, notably cricket and football, which were compulsory subjects at their public schools. Expending their energy outdoors during the day on the sports field in all-male peer company at the many sports clubs across the capital and its suburbs proved for the majority a more healthy exercise than being cramped inside stuffy London drawing rooms late at night, under the watchful eye of young women and their chaperones.

The English gentleman: codes of chivalry and manliness

In the eyes of Society matriarchs, dancing masters, etiquette writers, and many among the English bourgeoisie, the chivalrous actions of men towards women remained highly desirable. The medieval notion of chivalry had been revived in the late eighteenth century and developed as an ideal of masculinity that distinguished the English gentleman (Girouard, 1981). Commitment to unstintingly gallant and courteous behaviour towards women may have resembled the eighteenth-century code of politeness, but Victorian chivalry differed in the emphasis placed upon defending women, the empire, and civilization. The English gentleman of the nineteenth century should not only be ever ready to attend to the safety and comfort of women in social situations; he should also be prepared to leave her side to fight on her behalf and that of his sovereign and country. Over the course of the century, the domestic, social, and emotional sphere of Victorian women increasingly lost ground to the public arena of male thought and physical action. The code of chivalry was not solely responsible for this shift which brought together a complex and labile mix of ideological and material concerns with respect to the education and socialization of young males.

From the 1840s, the cult of manliness, though already present in eighteenth-century discourse, was especially cultivated within the public school sector. Manliness was constructed as the exclusive province of the English gentleman who typically displayed emotional reserve, courage, decisiveness, independence, strength, vigour, resolution, firmness, and straightforwardness (Mangan and Walvin, 1987; Tosh, 2005a). These were traits that might best be displayed on the sports or battlefield where men met men in a competitive environment; they were features less fitted to domestic drawing rooms or the ball room. Over the course of the century, the concept grew in popularity alongside and sometimes eclipsed in importance the earlier nineteenth-century revival of chivalric gallantry towards women. Manly ideals appeared more apposite to men of the British nation, whether battling long and hard on foreign fields, or in the financial offices that drove the empire. The cult of manliness also embraced a strong work ethic that was taken by many among the middle classes to set them apart from the aristocracy on social, economic, and moral grounds. Separate education, physical training in field sports, the military, the club, the work environment and, increasingly, leisure pursuits developed a male bonding that excluded women. In the debate over the shortage of men in the ball room, the intertwined discourses of chivalry and manliness were called upon by both critics and supporters of dancing men. As one critic thundered:

'When Nature built man she gave him an arm to wield a sword and a foot to tramp the world, but never a toe to trip with light and airy tread across the polished floor of a nineteenth century ball-room.'[19]

Not all were convinced by this imperialist bombast. One defender of dancing men retaliated that while the wallflowers languished, the missing men were more likely to be found playing 'the manly game of nap or billiards'.[20]

Fighting to protect male interest in dancing, Scott argued that the quality of manliness might be inculcated within the traditional fancy dance repertoire of boys; even though traditionally male-gendered dances such as the Jockey Dance, Irish Jig, and Sailor's Hornpipe, were mostly taught by and in the company of young women and, by the 1890s, were increasingly being exhibited by young girls. The Sailor's Hornpipe, however, had long held an exceptional place in popular affection as both a male and 'national dance par excellence' (Grove, 1895, p. 124; Bratton, 1990). Scott (1892, p. 114) enthused that the dance was 'distinctly *vigorous* and *manly* [original emphasis] ... in it animation, strength, and defiance alone are represented'. His characterization of the dance (1892, p. 113) blends notions of the work ethic, aristocratic self-possession, and imperialist supremacy as embodied national characteristics:

> [T]he folding of the arms in an attitude, not of laziness – remember that – but of conscious strength. The upper part of the body is kept in a state of calm repose, while the lower limbs are executing the most complicated, rapid, and difficult movements. Is not all this typical of an ideally English trait? To appear calm and collected amid circumstances calculated to induce a condition of physical and mental agitation.

Such attributes of collected calm, vigour, and manliness as essential qualities of English masculinity would reverberate into the next century and across other dance forms (see Chapter 17).

In the closing decade of the nineteenth century, a charge increasingly levelled at dancing men was the very antithesis of manliness: effeminacy. Contemporary meanings of effeminacy, however, did not typically bear the later connotations of homosexuality (Sinfield, 1994). Concurrent with earlier belief in gender as a socialization process rather than as a biological given, the Victorian interpretation of effeminacy suggested the weakening of men through too much time spent in female company (Cohen, 1996). In the polar construction of late nineteenth-century gender, male dancing, typically enjoyed with women, threatened culturally approved norms of virility and manliness. Furthermore, the eighteenth-century representation by political reformers and the rising bourgeoisie of the leisured aristocracy as effete and powerless (Kuchta, 1996) strengthened over the next century. Perceived as immoral and profligate, customary aristocratic life, with its many balls and conspicuous consumption, stood in opposition to typical middle-class values of temperance and sobriety. In the wake of the revolutions, Industrial, American, and French, dancing might be considered unmanly for male aristocrats, nervous of losing power and needing to be counted as working for nation and empire (Colley, 2005).

A long tradition of puritanical and middle-class opposition to the pleasures of the body and of time-wasting frivolity, contributed to the cultural status of dancing as an insignificant activity for the captains of British industry and empire. Following Cartesian thought, dancing, in late nineteenth-century neo-Romantic discourse, was typically viewed as an art of the body and as an expression of the emotions, rather than of the brain, and therefore, according to Victorian gendered norms, aligned with the female domain. Male dancing became increasingly positioned as being, in essence, more 'natural' for foreigners, especially the Latin races, who, in British xenophobic sentiment, were regarded as less able to contain emotional expression in voluble gesticulation (see Chapter 16). Even the language of dance – French – was that of the foreigner and, indeed, by the nineteenth century, a language similarly declining in British male approbation as Cohen (1996) has argued. French and dancing were now regarded as essentially female endeavours, ornamental and dispensable. Graceful dancing and correct deportment, 'la danse gracieuse' and 'bonne tenue' once the necessary accomplishments of royalty and aristocracy, had shifted towards the domain of the powerless, the female, and the childlike. It is perhaps no coincidence that in Victorian entertainment, dancing dogs, the epithet aimed at dancing men, were a show of little consequence, unnatural and amusing. Typically, dancing dogs were poodles, an elegant yet decorative French breed, defined in anti-French sentiment as oppositional to John Bull's stout and aggressive English terrier, which was bred for force rather than for grace.[21]

In the closing years of Victoria's reign, male interest in dancing at Society functions appeared to be submerged by a complex of interacting ideologies and events, the resulting wash of which was to promote recognition of dance as a female activity. In the seemingly quieter waters of the increasingly affluent and time-richer middle classes, however, older currents and fresh channels of dancing, springing up and flowing across from nearby and further abroad, were poised to carry away a new generation on a wave of enthusiasm of dancing. No longer channelled by the guardians of polite convention, but by the advocates of free flowing innovation, dancing swept both young women and young men into a turbulent sea of seemingly uncharted modernity.

Part III
Modern Moves

13
Moving into the Twentieth Century

[I]f we would not be left behind, we must march with
the times – and dance, with them, too.
George Grossmith in Naylor (1913), p. 230

At the beginning of the twentieth century, social dancing among the
higher echelons of British society was in a stagnated state. The repertoire,
little changed over several generations, was often executed out of a sense
of duty, particularly by Society men whose dwindling numbers in the
ball room had been yet more depleted by losses during the second Anglo-
Boer war (1899–1902). Ball-giving and attendance were further curtailed
when Victoria's death in 1901 plunged the nation into mourning. The
customary curb on public entertainment on the death of a monarch hon-
oured a queen who, although the majority of the population had never
seen her during her many reclusive years, was regarded as a symbol of the
permanence of Britain's imperial supremacy and of a way of life that was
essentially rule bound, morally conservative, and deferential in terms of
age, class, race, and gender.[1]

Edwardian England's Society dance culture maintained many of the
previous century's stalwart features. Young aristocratic women continued to 'come out' at the Season's private dances which were dominated
almost entirely by fast Waltzes, interspersed with a very occasional Two-
Step. Debutantes lined up in ever greater numbers at the Drawing Rooms
of the new monarchs as Society, described by one cynic, became 'open to
almost anyone who has a mind to enter it' (Pascoe in Evans and Evans,
1976, p. 11; see also Armytage, 1927). An increasingly prosperous lower-
middle class imitated the genteel ways of an earlier age in town halls
and hired rooms, at the dancing teacher assemblies on Friday, Saturday,
and some mid-week evenings. Here, the repertoire was more diverse even

though backward-looking. Waltzes were performed at a sedate pace, along-side various sets of Quadrilles and highly popular sequence dances such as the Veleta and Military Two-Step. Such ready-made choreographies suited the enthusiastic but deeply conservative clientele who followed the tenets of Victorian dance technique. Lower-middle-class dancers favoured the mix of security and novelty in the season's new dance combinations which had been approved, often in competitions, by professional pedagogic organizations at annual congresses.

But if Edward's reign appeared in many respects to be a continuation of high Victorian mores, undercurrents of modern social and artistic trends set in motion from the 1870s were gathering greater momentum. Former acquiescence in the old order began to totter visibly as the effects of faster communication, expanding educational opportunities, moves towards emancipation for women, widening prosperity, shifts in economic power, and greater political representation wrought lasting changes in both social relations and in public forms of expression. Strait-laced conventions of etiquette became increasingly dismissed as old-fashioned by a generation eager for more relaxed social interaction and cultural practices of a kind they felt to be more in tune with modern times.

Outside the stultified atmosphere of the state balls, the future of social dancing came to lie increasingly with the wealthy bourgeoisie, who together with dance-loving Society members, embraced a new world of sound and relative social freedom in the ballroom. By the end of the first decade, social dancing among the upper bourgeoisie was transformed from the staid conventions of a hierarchical, private and conservative Victorian dance culture to that of a democratic, public, and innovative scene, where demand for novelty and celebrity, in an increasingly consumerist society, endorsed the publications of a growing influential media.

By the early twentieth century, the chaperone system at Society balls and dances was well in abeyance. It still lingered in a few traditionalist strongholds even after the First World War, as the young daughters of families at court continued to be cocooned away from experiences of the greater physical and social freedoms enjoyed by their bourgeois sisters. Although aristocrats, such as Lady Manners who was reputed to be the greatest beauty of her age, and royal women, particularly the queens Alexandra and Mary, were looked to as models of fashion and deportment for upper- and middle-class women, stage celebrities and dancers were increasingly profiled in the press as modern exemplars of womanhood. Youth, vitality, natural beauty, and a slim less-corseted physique were markers of a fresh ideal of femininity; and in dancing socially and artistically, such 'modern' women were to seek and appreciate less restrained ways of moving as they approached the new century.

By the end of the first decade, the old, uniform circling around the dance floor and sedately paced Quadrilles to European flowing melodies had been abandoned by the young and fashionable in favour of musical and choreographic influences from across the Atlantic. The new rhythms and accompanying movements caused many of the older generation to click their tongues in disapproval and lament the yet further decline of civilization as young couples hugged one another on the public dance floor, improvising to the syncopated rhythms of ragtime, or swaying in the intimate contact of the Argentine Tango. Widespread questioning of long accepted social behaviour, together with a renaissance of interest in dance, both as professional entertainment to be watched and as recreation, came to a crescendo in the four years before the outbreak of the First World War. This sense of restless vitality, hedonism and search for novelty dovetailed with what was widely regarded as the end of the old order. George V's accession in 1910 was hailed as a new era of modernity, even if in reality the new king was ultra-conservative in his insistence on observing protocol and tradition. George and his queen Mary stuck rigidly to the old regime of Waltzes and Quadrilles while younger, more fun-seeking members of their court enjoyed the thrilling music and movement of London's fast-expanding restaurant culture and nightclubs.

During this period of revitalization, the fashionable social dance repertoire can broadly be divided into three categories, based on the criteria of each dance's supposed provenance and choreographic characteristics. First are those dances already familiar from the nineteenth century which had undergone transformations in the ballroom, the most notable of these being the Waltz in its guise as the Boston. Second are the ragtime dances, transported from North America, which are distinguished by syncopated rhythms and comparative simplicity of movement vocabulary, a classic example being the One-Step. Third and finally are the more complex dances of Latin America, epitomized by the Argentine Tango. These categories, however, are by no means watertight; indeed, a distinguishing feature of the dance culture of this period is its highly labile and hybrid nature, indicative not only of the complex and swiftly changing times, but also married to a new insistence on the freedom to improvise and the right to express the self.

The dancing of the upper bourgeoisie

Early in Edward's reign, a distinctive social group of dedicated dancers became apparent in central London and its near suburbs. These wealthy young dancers were able to take advantage of the privileges of more time and space in new public venues to advance their technique, often nightly in the individualistic and improvisational manner that the inchoate repertoire afforded them. A renaissance in social dancing was to take hold across the country, but the infrastructure for the 'shock of the new' that was to instigate outcries of horror and disapproval from the establishment in the years prior to the First World War was quietly being laid in these days of the seeming doldrums. Where the much desired improvements in social dancing emerged they were not manifest among Society, but in the public, yet still exclusive, dance gatherings of the upper bourgeoisie.

When the revived *Dancing Times* reported in its first issue of 1910 that the regular series of subscription dances organized by suburban sports clubs were declining in steady patronage, the blame could not be laid at the familiar door of lack of interest in dancing; quite the contrary. The well-to-do with a mind to dance were being attracted in large numbers to the more sophisticated subscription dance series on offer in the function rooms of the fashionable quarters of south-west London and the West End.[2] Excellent bus, underground, tram, and train routes facilitated ready evening access to the city centre from the suburbs, bringing a smart professional class to dine and to dance in a manner quite impossible in most middle-class private homes. The Carlton Rooms, the Grafton Galleries, and the opulent ballrooms of the newly built large hotels attracted a glamorous crowd of minor aristocracy and upper bourgeoisie to its subscription series where the young and dedicated were eager to acquire and to hone a repertoire that reflected their cultural values. Mainly disassociated from the direct control of teachers, unfettered by the old-fashioned chaperone system and unpoliced by Society matriarchs, the subscription dances of the upper-middle class marked a growing yet respectable freedom of relations between the sexes, an interest in embracing social dancing as pleasurable leisure rather than social duty and the congregation of like-minded people to pursue their interest.

Enthusiasts from Society and the upper bourgeoisie began to meet regularly as a dancing club in these attractive new venues, sometimes several nights a week. In central London, the most well-patronized were the Royalist Club, founded in 1910 at the Connaught Rooms (Great Queen Street) which then housed the largest permanent dance floor in the capital and the Public Schools and Universities Dance Club established at the Savoy Hotel in 1911.[3] These organizations were clubs in the sense that they were open to private membership on payment of an annual subscription, but their premises were not purpose built, nor did the club necessarily patronize only one establishment at a time.

New ways of waltzing

Dances favoured by the clientele in 1910 were occasional Two-Steps, the newer One-Step to American ragtime melodies and the Boston, performed to the fresh music of the English school of waltz composers. Foremost among these dances in the early 1900s was the Boston. Although performed to waltz music, in essence the Boston heralded a radical departure from the Victorian rotary form of Waltz. Gone were the neat steps derived from balletic positions of the feet in favour of a more naturalistic means of progression. To the undiscerning eye, such movement suggested an eschewal of technique, appearing akin to ordinary walking. But in reality, competence in this method of waltzing required specific skills that were the result of frequent practice on spacious, smooth floors. Contrary to the criticisms of its detractors (see Figure 13.1), of whom there were later to be many, when danced well, the Boston was an emblem of refined dancing: smooth, gracious, and a perfect vehicle to display skill and distinction.

The route of the Boston into fashionable London ballrooms was mainly via the sophisticated seaside resorts of northern France, such as Dinard, Trouville, Deauville, and Le Touquet, frequented by Parisians, aristocratic

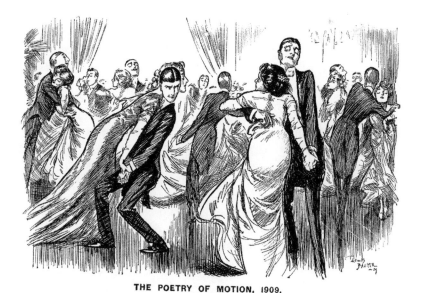

THE POETRY OF MOTION, 1909.
The " Boston."

Figure 13.1   The Poetry of Motion, *Punch*, 17 February 1909

Europeans, and rich Americans during the summer months. Small wonder then that the Boston became the favoured waltz style of the fashionable select: only they frequented the smart hotel and casino circuit of European resorts, and had both time and money to spend in perfecting their technique in the equivalent venues of London's West End hotels.

From the early 1900s, a dedicated band of Boston enthusiasts had begun to meet regularly at the Empress Rooms in the Royal Palace Hotel in Kensington.[4] Organized by Miss Janet Lennard, this series of subscription dances afforded a regular opportunity for practice and enjoyment. Known as the Keen Dancers Society or K. D. S., the group of dancers met at a number of venues before re-naming itself the Boston Club which Janet Lennard and Mrs Picton Ellett ran at the Grafton Galleries. It was through this association of Boston lovers that subsequent developments in social dancing were frequently introduced from the continent, to be endorsed and shaped for later emulation by fashionable society. Other dedicated dance clubs that favoured the Boston over the traditional Waltz emerged in the London suburbs of Hampstead, Ealing, Blackheath, and Croydon.[5] It was in these venues that a committed following for innovative ways of dancing became socially acceptable, ushering in a new focus on dance as a leisure activity and, in the process, raising the standard of performance.

The Boston had its devotees and its detractors, not exactly in equal measure, as some dancers were perfectly capable of performing both this new dance and the older Waltz. Both forms were executed to waltz music and it was this continuity of musical rhythm that eased the Boston's comparatively quiet acceptance onto the early Edwardian dance floor. Confusion over what constituted the Boston was evident in press coverage at the end of the first decade, but few newspaper testimonies were drawn from firsthand knowledge. Even among established dancing teachers and Boston practitioners, there was dissent as to the dance's precise rendition and character. Some considered it to be an American variation on the Waltz that had been popular around the 1870s; others argued that it was an entirely new form that had arisen on the continent. Some pronounced it a recent strategy to maintain balance and breath when attempting to waltz to the increasingly fast pace of the German bands. And yet others dismissed it as nothing more than bad dancing by people who were unable to waltz properly. Such division of opinion is characteristic of the emergence of a new mode of dancing, and elements of truth no doubt lay in each of these depictions.[6]

Some features were, however, relatively consistent: the adoption of the American or Boston hold in which partners positioned themselves hip to hip while facing each other; the use of parallel rather than turned out feet; the travelling around the floor employing gliding long steps on the whole foot, rather than stepping neatly toe first and rising onto the balls of the feet on the turn, as in the traditional Waltz step. Allied to this, the even pace of the Boston steps was far more akin to walking than to the dactylic – *u u* rhythm of the Victorian Waltz step, and it enabled a more leisurely tenor to be maintained throughout the dance. The fact that the dancers executed one complete turn over four bars of music rather than the Waltz's two underlined the Boston's distinctive use of space. The Boston was essentially a linear dance, whereas the waltz was rotary.

The Victorian ball room ideal resided in the symmetry of spinning couples, all evenly positioned and turning around the edges of the ball room. The Boston broke this choreographic uniformity. Instead, the Boston couple orientated themselves on a diagonal angle to the line of dance. The man gently propelled his partner backwards on a straight line towards the centre of the room, an area avoided by traditional waltzers. Having reached a point close to the room's centre, he might then decide to guide his partner back toward the outer wall of the room, moving forwards on a diagonal. This zig-zag manner of progression, however, posed a threat to the harmony of the ballroom.

Opportunities for collision were rife as couples performing the Boston and the Waltz treated space and time differently: although both progressed counter-clockwise around the room, they did so at different speeds and using different spatial trajectories. Added to this, the rotary waltzer had limited options to get himself and his partner out of possible harm. His only real options were to vary the speed of progression or to stop dancing completely and get out of the way of oncoming dancers. The expert Boston dancer, on the other hand, armed with a greater variety of manoeuvres, might shepherd his partner away from potential hazard by the judicious selection of dance steps that could move them onto safe ground, without breaking the flow of the routine. Responding to likely impediments to smooth progress in the room, he might turn his partner into a new direction, or select steps such as the 'crab', to take them sideways, or the 'run' to progress them further away from an advancing couple. Judgement and quick decision-making was called for on the dance floor, requiring practice to cultivate the necessary skills.

Despite its growing popularity among the upper-middle classes in London, the Boston continued to be condemned by many Victorian waltzers. The appeal of a freer music-dance association in the Boston, so attractive to its practitioners, was regarded as anathema to the traditionalists.

Whereas the latter ideally transferred their weight with each step to the three beats of one bar of music, the Boston dancers moved across the musical bar, responding to the melody. In the traditionalists' eyes, this signalled unmusical dancing. For the Boston dancer, it resulted in a sensation akin to skating, especially when dancers moved to a swinging melody by one of the new school of English composers, such as 'Dreaming' by Archibald Joyce (1911) or 'Destiny' by Sydney Baynes (1912).[7]

Regardless of censure, the Boston continued to thrive in its myriad manifestations up to the beginning of the First World War. New variations christened the 'Double' and the 'Triple' Boston gained the most acceptance and the dance was a regular feature in the advertisements of most up-to-the minute London dancing-teachers' classes. Walter Humphrey (1911b) and Janet Lennard (1911) contributed on the Boston to the *Dancing Times*, the Imperial Society of Dance Teachers provided advice on its correct execution in their *Dance Journal* and even Edward Scott (1913) devoted a whole monograph to the dance; though experienced Boston dancer, Philip Richardson, was not convinced that the Victorian dancing master had thoroughly grasped its essential character.[8] For the dancer to experience the skating sensation, its execution required not only the correct positioning of the feet and hold, but a new length of step that swung from the hip and shoulder, prefiguring a key element in the distinctive English style of ballroom dancing that was to be refined in the 1920s and 1930s.

14
Modernizing Terpsichore

> We know that anything bizarre or unexpected is apt to
> fascinate the present day generation.
>
> *The Dancing Times*, December 1912, p. 134

While fashionable dancers were experimenting with new moves in the ballroom, the commercial realm of the popular theatre eagerly sought dance novelties for its growing audiences. By 1908, newspapers were celebrating a dance renaissance on the British stage.[1] In several respects, the new vogue for dancing could be considered reflective, symptomatic, and emblematic of the sense of modernity evident across many discourses, especially in art, literature, music, politics, science, and technology, at the turn of the twentieth century. The sense of gathering pace, the desire for new aural and spectacular sensations, the search for a *frisson* of the exotic, increasing mobility both socially and geographically and the expansion of a more prosperous and leisured population contributed to a self-conscious desire among many to align themselves with what were regarded as distinctly 'modern' cultural practices.

Exhibiting the latest dance sensations

Sixty years before, the Polka sensation had demonstrated the commercial and cultural capital of novel dance forms; the late-nineteenth-century expansion in theatres, the press and transport presented perfect conditions for the marketing of new dances which were channelled and legitimated through a much changed but still culturally authoritative Paris. The French capital held the palm in the British collective imagination as the 'quintessence of modernity' (Tombs and Tombs, 2006, p. 373) as well as signalling the ultimate destination for the traveller, usually male, intent on pursuing hedonism and vice. The Prince of Wales, irreverently referred to at home as 'Edward the Caresser', was notoriously known to be familiar with Parisian delights of the eye and flesh. In the later nineteenth century, the French capital, acknowledged for centuries as the refined cultural leader of Europe, had been remarketed as 'gay Paree', the haunt of many a wealthy young man out on the town. Although Paris would continue a centuries-old reputation for sophistication and taste, its many new or revivified bars, cafés, and public dance halls, notably in the Bohemian district of Montmartre, encouraged an innovative culture of daring experimentation in the arts, as well as promoting far more relaxed social mores than might be found in London Society. In addition to its dissolute reputation, Paris was a comparatively cheap European city in which to live, as testified by the numbers of émigrés, impoverished aristocracy, bankrupts, and artists resident in the capital. It was also the first stop for many transatlantic passengers on the European tour, an attraction for rich North Americans and wealthy Argentinean émigrés, many of whom frequented the glamorous Café de Paris and Maxim's. These venues, together with Parisian salons, the hotel restaurants and ballrooms of France's northern and southern rivieras, were to be of considerable significance in the development of exhibition ballroom dancing that swept Europe and North America from the 1910s.[2]

London may have trailed behind Paris in fostering innovative and liberal public performances, yet by the early 1900s, the face of public evening entertainment in London had changed considerably. At the Gaiety Theatre, home of the newly evolving musical comedy, reputable women as well as men turned out to view the spectacle of fashionable yet modest femininity presented by the Gaiety Girls. Music halls, once shunned by respectable men and their families, had become gentrified into capacious theatres of comfort and good reputation, attracting the ranks of the affluent middle classes. At new, revamped and often re-licensed theatres such as the London Hippodrome, the Empire, the Palace, the Alhambra, and Princes, proprietors took advantage of the Music Hall Licensing Act to include dancing on their stages.[3] Restaurants attached to or close by West End theatres, such as the Savoy, the Criterion, the Cecil and the Carlton Hotel restaurants drew a wealthy clientele who might now bring their wives, rather than their mistresses, to dine. Noting the improvement in music-hall entertainment over the last ten to fifteen years, the 1908 Baedeker guide to London advised that 'ladies may visit the better-class West End establishments without fear, although they should, of course, eschew the cheaper seats'. During the day, middle- and upper-class ladies were visible on the smarter streets of London, shopping, taking tea, and attending the recently instituted theatre matinées (see Rappaport, 2001). Theatre and music-hall proprietors competitively sought high-class yet novel dance acts to appeal to their new audiences, catering for the growing public fascination with watching dancing. Stage celebrities graced the pages of Society and the popular press alongside or even overshadowing aristocracy as iconic leaders of taste.[4]

Contrasting the fecundity of theatre dance with the barren ballroom, the Edwardian press scrutinized the various dance acts for potential transferral to the social dance floor.[5] An initial candidate was the Cake Walk, the first African-American dance to be entertained by white society as an entrant to the Euro-American ball room canon. The Cake Walk was already familiar to audiences of British music-hall stages in the late 1890s from blackface minstrelsy and theatre scenes depicting supposed plantation life. Sheet music illustrations further cemented the connection as did the hugely popular performances of Leslie Stuart's song 'The Cake Walk' by Eugene Stratton, the blackface entertainer in 1898. Indeed, so strong was the perceived association between the Cake Walk and racist theatricalized depictions of African-American culture that when the first all-black musical theatre show *In Dahomey* played at the Shaftesbury Theatre in London in 1903, audiences demanded that the stereotypical dance be inserted into the production.[6]

The Cake Walk was not favoured in the ballroom, however, in spite of its Parisian success and promotion by American composer John Philip Sousa on his European tour. To its syncopated march accompaniment, partners moved shoulder to shoulder, each couple facing the line of dance, free to improvise on an individual basis. Its hallmarks were a strutting high-stepping walk, the body leaning backwards, both arms lifted in front of the chest and bent at the elbow, with the wrists bent and hands limp. The dance seems to have enjoyed some popularity in Lancashire (Richardson, 1960) and at 'shilling hops' in London. Even at the latter, however, Robert Machray observed a certain reluctance among dancers to engage in the dance, possibly, he speculated, because it required 'so much abandon' or because it was 'so complete a caricature of Turvey-dropism' (1902, p. 159). The fact that the dance achieved a modicum of acceptance by groups far from the centre of aristocratic power – dancers in the north and from the lower-middle classes – might support a thesis of subaltern mockery of the upper and London-centred classes. The Cake Walk, however, had an earlier existence in black slave caricature of the plantation owners' dancing of the Minuet and March Round the Ball Room (see Stearns and Stearns, 1968); small wonder that it did not appeal to British polite society to perform themselves, however faint the echoes of mockery. Regardless of understanding of the dance's likely origins in covert satire, the Cake Walk's contemporary affiliation to a musical and dance culture regarded as primitive (see Chapter 16) was likely to be sufficient reason to dissuade most white dancers from its imitation. To appeal to white middle- and upper-class dancers, future importations would need to be more thoroughly mediated through white bodies, both in terms of kinetic style and representation. This was a role upon which music-hall entertainers and, later, exhibition ballroom dancers in restaurants and theatres would capitalize.

Dance acts had long featured as popular entertainment in Britain, but with the rise of musical comedy and the romantic operetta, there appeared to be a fresh focus upon heterosexual couple dancing. In 1905, for example, French dancer, composer and choreographer Camille De Rhynal performed a Brazilian Maxixe (Richardson, 1946) with rising star Gabrielle Ray at the Prince of Wales Theatre in the musical comedy *Lady Madcap*, produced by George Edwardes. Two years later, De Rhynal sought to follow this up with another, but far more sultry, South American import for Edwardes, the Argentine Tango. Despite its perceived potential, the dance in its existing guise was not considered suitable for London theatre audiences (Silvester and Richardson, 1936) who were known to be far more prudish than their Parisian counterparts. Several more years of 'refinement', adoption by the international smart set and shifts in English boundaries of taste were to occur before the Tango was successfully introduced onto the London stage.

Meanwhile, the Waltz remained a familiar dance rhythm on the British stage. Even this staple was given fresh inflection in the early 1900s, most notably in two contrasting depictions of heterosexual passion. The first was the Waltz in the hugely popular Viennese operetta *The Merry Widow* by Franz Lehar, produced by George Edwardes in London in 1907. Here, a dreamy, languorous waltz was employed to reveal the hidden depth of tender love between its aristocratic leads within the sophisticated context of Austro-Hungarian embassy life in Paris. Such an interpretation of upper-class romance was logical enough given the dance's nineteenth-century history as a dance of courtship among the well-to-do.

Far more radical renderings of the Waltz were French music-hall star Gaby Deslys's Ju Jitsu Waltz performed with a martial art expert at the Gaiety Theatre in the same year and, even more acrobatic and combative, the Apache Waltz.[7] This latter was a theatricalized representation of male-female relations in gangland Paris. It had been popularised by French music-hall artists Max Dearly and Mistinguett who, in her role of the physically and emotionally abused girl, reputedly 'brought into the dance all the nervous excitement of modernity' (Flitch, 1912, p. 183). Introduced by British dancers Fred Farren and Beatrice Collier in the Empire production *A Day in Paris* in 1908, the violence and athleticism of the Apache dance was testimony to the appeal of the exotic 'other' which, in this instance, was located for the sedate British middle class and Society audiences in the imagined spheres of the uncivilized underclass in the shocking city of Paris (Tickner, 2000). The dance act remained a popular variety spectacle for several decades under the new name of adagio dancing, while its stereotypical characters – he distinguishable by his rough clothes, cap, kerchief, and cigarette and she by her short slit skirt, tight blouse, and beret – proved staple fancy dress characters at early twentieth-century balls. The Apache Waltz, not surprisingly, given its many lifts and throws was not at all appropriate for the ballroom, but its appearance on the London stage in 1908 marked a distinctive shift in the 'tone and feeling' of dancing.[8] The scene was set for a more permissible range of proxemics, dynamics, and experimentation.

On the continent, in smart cafés and hotel restaurants, managers were hiring theatrical dance acts as part of the cabaret for their wealthy diners. One of the earliest proponents of this vogue, who was to lead internationally in crossing the line between the stage and social dance floor, was Maurice Mouvet (1889–1927), an American born of Belgian parents who, as a young boy, was educated in England before moving to Paris. During his teenage years he watched the dancing at Maxim's from the doorway; the images of privilege and glamour were ones that he would later reflect back to his rich clientele. Mouvet reputedly acquired his technique through observation and imitation, initially of the African-American dancers performing the Cake Walk at the Nouveau Cirque café in Paris. He was hired as a solo dancer, later partnering in the 'dance teams' in Montmartre, before he learned to waltz at afternoon dances at the Bal Tabarin (Mouvet, [1915]). Following engagements at the Café Royale, the Casino Theatre, Vienna (where he learned the famous Viennese rapid style of waltzing), the Park Theatre, Budapest, the Carlton Hotel in Monte Carlo, and the Café de Paris, Maurice, as he was later to be most famously known, performed before and taught aristocrats, international celebrities and the moneyed in Parisian salons, before arriving in New York in October 1910 to dance at Louis Martin's restaurant. Here, Maurice performed the Argentine Tango and Apache dance, the latter speciality acquired, according to his autobiography, from the dance's original practitioners in the caverns of lowlife Paris.

Mouvet's place at the Café de Paris was later to be taken by the Anglo-American husband-and-wife partnership Vernon and Irene Castle who, on their return to the United States in 1912, became his greatest rivals.[9] Between them, Mouvet and the Castles were regarded as the leading exponents of exhibition ballroom dancing, but both had secured success through testing their mettle in the crucible of high society Parisian entertainment. The Castles' publicity machine was to overshadow the role of many other exhibition ballroom dancers and teachers in refining the new repertoire. In Britain, it was in fact Maurice's elder brother Oscar whom Philip Richardson was to praise as the 'most graceful ballroom dancer I have ever seen'.[10] Engaged at the Hippodrome Theatre in 1912, Oscar and his partner, Suzette, were among the first of the exhibition ballroom dancers to excite London audiences to imitate their style and repertoire. Included in their act was the infamous ragtime dance, the Turkey Trot, regarded by many social commentators as indicative of a worrying descent from the ideals of civilized behaviour.[11] But disquiet over terpsichorean standards on stage had already been voiced. A *Times* review of the 1909 production of *The Merry Widow*, worried that, since the introduction of the Apache, some theatrical dancing had a 'tendency to neglect what is beautiful in the art for a feature which we should be very sorry to see introduced into our ballrooms'.[12] Established notions of the beautiful in dancing were about to be swept away as American ragtime and its associated animal dances flooded onto the popular stage and into fashionable European ballrooms. Widely popularized through musical revues and piano sheet music, London's enthusiasm for ragtime in Britain peaked in responses to the long running show, *Hullo Ragtime*. The first of several imports from New York, based on Parisian-style musical revues, the production was introduced by Albert de Courville at the Hippodrome, featuring American artists such as Shirley Kellogg and Ethel Levey. The show included early Irving Berlin numbers such as 'Hitchy Koo', 'Alexander's Ragtime Band' and 'Everybody's Doing It,' the latter's lyrics urging the stage characters and by implication the audience to join in dancing to the intoxicating music.

Teaching the new repertoire

Initially, no English dynasties in the dance pedagogic profession capitalized upon the new trends in social dancing. It was left to enthusiasts such as Janet Lennard of the K. D. S. Daughter of a shipowner and resident in London's West End, she was one of a growing breed of dance instructors who, unlike the generalist teachers of the Victorian era, focused almost entirely upon fashionable social dancing and whose circle was the upper-middle classes. There were, however, a few open-minded and entrepreneurial established dancing teachers who recognized the exigencies of change. Recurring names of West End teachers offering classes in the new dances were predominantly female: in addition to Janet Lennard were Madame Alice Vandyck, Miss Janet Thomas, and Miss Marguerite Vacani, later to take the palm of royal tutelage away from Louis D'Egville and from Mrs Wordsworth.[13]

Around 1901, Walter Humphrey of the London Academy of Dancing sought out a former pupil at the Empress Rooms at the Royal Palace Hotel, Kensington. Prompted by demand from his own upper-middle-class pupils, Humphrey recognized the need to learn the Boston himself in order to stay abreast of changing fashion. On trips to Paris, he acquired new styles of dancing, often authenticating his own transmission through reference to well-known continental teachers. In the early issues of the newly re-launched *Dancing Times*, in addition to the latest and most correct mode of dancing the Boston, he wrote on the recent ragtime introductions of the One-Step and earlier Two-Step and advised on a leading article on Tango. Humphrey retained his high ranking as specialist teacher and advisor to *The Dancing Times* during the pre-war craze for the new ballroom dances, even though his authority was not monolithic or indeed unchallenged.[14]

Annual waves of new dances brought forth many new claimants to the profession of dance teaching as public appetite to learn the fresh repertoire expanded. Entertainment in the new restaurant culture effected considerable change in the dance pedagogic profession. Instead of attending assemblies at dancing academies on a regular basis as in the past, the affluent public could now learn the new dance repertoire as they dined in hotels and restaurants. Exhibitions by international performers in high-class restaurants opened opportunities for dancers to give private instruction in the homes of very rich clients and in public venues such as the music hall and theatre. Especially popular in the dancing season of 1912–13 were the *thés dansants* or tango teas, as they were popularly known in Britain, where dancing could be learned as part of a social event in the late afternoon (see Chapter 15). Exhibition dancers entertained the observers with displays of the latest dances and variations before doubling up as teachers. A differential price was charged for those watching and for those wishing to learn from the exhibition dancers and their assistants. Stellar exhibition couples such as Oscar and Suzette, Maurice Mouvet and Florence Walton, Los Almanos and, most famous of all, America-based Irene and Vernon Castle had little time to provide regular personal tuition to large numbers of the British population anxious to learn the dances. Most restricted their private classes to aristocratic and wealthy clienteles, or to the dance teaching profession.

At the height of the Tango craze in the season of 1912–13, demand for exhibition dancers threatened to exceed supply.[15] Theatrical styles of dancing, transferred without adaptation to the ballroom, had always been regarded with disapproval by Society and by reputable instructors; but the public hunger to see and learn African-American sourced dances, as well as other ballroom dances such as the Waltz, had not been matched by any widespread positive response from the established pedagogic profession. An initial problem was that the public wanted to learn the new dances quickly and tried to do so by imitating the often showy and acrobatic routines of the musical theatre and music hall. Where tuition was available, it was often provided by performers without pedagogic competence. In a complaint remarkably similar to that of Crompton and his colleagues over 20 years earlier, Philip Richardson lamented the sudden increase of '[a]ll sorts and conditions of people, from bar tenders to railway servants', whose amateur performances of the Tango and Maxixe enabled them to acquire a professional performance booking, but who then mistakenly believed that they could teach.[16] He was not alone in condemning such lack of professionalism.

Many of the new performers had served neither a lengthy apprenticeship as an articled pupil teacher, nor trodden the boards of the opera houses; yet they quickly infiltrated the ranks of the dance-teaching profession in response to public demand. Their expertise was accredited in the public's eye through regular appearances on continental and transatlantic tours, and performances in the smartest restaurants, ballrooms, theatres, and private salons of fashionable society; not through years of training under the mentorship of a long-established Society teacher. Dismissed as old-fashioned, those teachers who maintained a courtly clientele could afford to reject the new repertoire; but those young, adaptable, and entrepreneurial enough to respond to the new music and way of moving, added dances such as the Boston, the One-Step, and Tango to their advertisements. Thus, the impact of the new repertoire was not detrimental to the livelihood of every established teacher. Indeed, the sight of celebrity dancers at hotel and restaurant ballrooms often encouraged pupils to contact their local dancing academies for tuition in the new dances.[17]

Among the names of established teachers, however, one bears singling out: Belle Harding. Trained, like Walter Humphrey, in Victorian styles of movement, Isabella Harding (1866–1945) not only quickly adapted to the new dance repertoire but became a foremost exponent and influential disseminator of the latest dance fashions among a wider society. Early in her long teaching career, Harding had demonstrated considerable ambition and opportunism. Born in Ulverston, a north-west market town at the gateway to the Lake District, by her early twenties she had already made contact with the national and international circuit of social dance tuition and practice. She employed an assistant teacher, performed at Society drawing rooms with Robert Crompton, and travelled on her own initiative to Leipzig to be present at the 1892 Congress of German dancing masters, as the sole English representative. En route to the conference, she attended a casino ball in Ostende, and from the description in her letter to *Dancing* would seem already to be a seasoned traveller, familiar with the dancing habits of Dieppe, Boulogne, and Wiesbaden.[18]

In the years immediately preceding the First World War, Harding capitalized upon the new developments in dancing repertoire which, coupled with her dedication, tremendous capacity for hard work and enthusiasm, made her a minor celebrity and highly esteemed teacher in England. Richardson credited her as the first English teacher to introduce the wider British public to the French fashion for *thés dansants*.[19] Her spring programme for 1914 included the Ralli-Boston Club at the Empress Rooms on Mondays, a *Thé Dansant* Tango and Boston Club in the afternoon on Tuesdays, and children's classes in fancy dancing, classical, and national. She also offered instruction in court presentation and in Scotch reels, the latter no doubt for anyone wishing to attend the summer Caledonian Ball or who had received an invitation to travel north to Scotland for the early autumn balls. Richardson sang her praises as a 'splendid hostess' following the September holiday week of dance teaching and competitions held at the Hermitage and Atlantic hotels in Le Touquet, and two years later proclaimed that there was 'no teacher probably more widely known' (see Figure 14.1).[20]

Her success owed much to her initiative in implementing a rapid and country-wide system of dance training, together with a dance-event provision that catered for the well-to-do urban middle classes. Keen to learn the new dances, the smart and aspirant followers of fashion in Britain's metropolitan centres flocked to the grand hotels where Harding organized weekend courses and dances. From her winter headquarters in the Empress Rooms at the Royal Palace Hotel in Kensington, she extended her empire across the British Isles, providing tuition and dances in the best hotels of Brighton, Eastbourne, Scarborough, Birmingham, Edinburgh, Glasgow, and Cork. Her summer headquarters came to be located in the new northern French resort of Le Touquet just before the

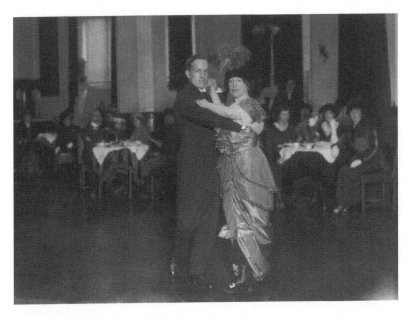

Figure 14.1 Society Tango, Belle Harding and partner

First World War, with centres in Paris, Le Hague, and Nice among others. Always alert to new leisure initiatives, from her 'Tours department' at the Empress Rooms, she even organized 'dancing holidays,' offering winter sports holiday packages to Grunewald in Switzerland.[21]

To maintain and meet the demand for instruction in Great Britain, Holland, and France, Harding needed to recruit a plentiful supply of trainee teachers. Her tactics were to play on middle-class concern to find suitable employment for their unmarried daughters. Heading her advertisements 'What to do with our Girls', Harding appealed to both the financial and social ambitions of parents, ensuring that she attracted the sort of clientele that could mix in good society and be prepared to pay for the privilege. Perhaps unusually she offered business training, guaranteed a position on completion (no doubt in one of her own centres), and tempted recruits with the possibility of training partially in Paris or The Hague.[22]

From her stable came the next generation's formative ballroom dance stylists, Georges Fontana and, most famously, Victor Silvester. In his autobiography, Silvester recalled the speed at which he was recruited as a temporary teacher for Harding soon after the end of the First World War. Taught by one of the 35 female student teachers Harding employed, he was judged after just two weeks to be sufficiently proficient to instruct the rich clients who came to the Empress Rooms. Earning a shilling per lesson (for which a client reputedly paid Belle Harding almost nine times as much), Silvester finally parted company with his employer when she refused to allow him to work on his day off at the rival Ritz Hotel. As a man, Silvester's experiences (Silvester, 1958) are not necessarily typical of most of Harding's pupil teachers; the young women were required to teach a far greater range of material including deportment and court presentation.

The hallmark of Harding's methods, like those of Mrs Wordsworth, relied upon a modernized version of the Victorian monitor system. What she lacked in fashionable youth and Society background, she compensated for with at least 20 years' experience of teaching dancing, long-established contact with the pedagogic profession on the European continent, and familiarity with its resort culture. She also possessed a sharp eye for dance novelties likely to appeal to the English, an organizational flair and understanding of publicity, effective management control of her staff, and an appreciation of new leisure trends among the middle class. Even the reversal of the ballet's status among the British aristocracy, consequent upon the arrival of the Ballets Russes in Paris and London, was seized upon as an opportunity by Belle Harding. Ever keen to be at the forefront of fashion, in her forties she became a pupil of Mikhail Mordkin, the famed danseur with Diaghilev's company and partner of Pavlova, and offered ballet as part of her courses. She even prospered during the war years, running charity dances, competitions, and classes for women and children at the Waldorf and Empress Rooms, while legally able under wartime restrictions, securing yet stronger foundations for when the public might renew its passion for dancing in peacetime.[23]

15
Civilization Under Threat

Since civilization will not teach us how to express our-
selves in art we are beginning to learn from barbarism.
'The Moral of the "Turkey Trot"', *The Times*,
26 May 1913

In the years preceding the First World War, widespread enthusiasm
for American musical and choreographic practices greatly unsettled
Victorian ideals of the 'ball room' as a microcosm of civilization. In the
perplexed and outraged eyes of the establishment, the once unchanging social hierarchy no longer reflected the modern 'ballroom'. Society
dance events were failing to function as showcases for the enactment
of corporeal balance, proportion, and grace, for the demonstration of
taste and manners at the highest level, and as models for strict control
of bodily spatial relations between the sexes. The Boston, the ragtime
dances, and the Tango, critics averred, transgressed all of these hallowed
social, moral, and aesthetic linchpins of Society dancing.

Ragging the dance

The new social dance repertoire was strongly influenced by African-
American rhythms, proxemics, and movement. Having evolved among
working-class, immigrant, and black neighbourhoods of urban America,
this dance material had been fashioned in theatre, music hall, ballroom,
and studio to appeal to a wider, mostly white spectatorship and participatory audience (see Berlin, 1980; Robinson, 2004, 2009, 2010). Via the
salons, cabarets, theatres, and hotels of fashionable France, this rapidly
changing repertoire of dances was embraced by a younger fashionable

160

generation in London which was keen to identify, not with the customs of their parents and grandparents, but with the innovative and shocking.

A run of new dances was offered to the general public by venue promoters, stage celebrities, the music industry, and the press who, for a while, overtook the traditional control of the pedagogic profession.[1] The new repertoire was eagerly sought by the young for it offered thrilling physical sensations of close bodily contact, driving ruptured rhythms, shockingly jerky movement, and the freedom to express individual personality on the dance floor. The public wanted sensations that were immediate, innovative, and indicative of an individual's ability to access *le denier cri* in cultural capital. Familiarity with the new distinguished the entrepreneurial, the individual within the ever greater urban crowd. In a modern sensibility, change not tradition was prized. The display of taste in music and dancing seemed more than ever to reflect the mark of sophistication achieved through personal effort and aptitude, rather than through the erstwhile privileges of birth, in a growing mass market where individual choices might be made.

Ragtime and Latin American dances were also showcased in theatres and restaurants by the new breed of exhibition dancers (Erenberg, 1981; Malnig, 1992, 2009a), a number of whom built performance and teaching careers for themselves out of their talent for social dancing.[2] Traditional routes and class expectations were often bypassed by a generation eager to shed the shackles of convention and to grasp the opportunities which a flourishing entertainment industry now brought. Many, nonetheless, did shift from the chorus line to centre stage (Malnig, 1992) and, as Philip Richardson approvingly noted at the time, manifested a training in operatic technique which, to his eye, rendered their performances more graceful and pleasing.[3]

In the ballroom, ragtime contrasted with the Boston's smooth progress through space; it emphasized a more staccato response to the music and required less practice to perfect the moves. It was a style of dancing that appealed to a generation keen to demonstrate itself to be in the latest fashion: easily imitated without the need for teachers, shocking in its aesthetics, in its challenge to social propriety, and overtly modern. The syncopated exuberance of African-American music evident in the Cake Walk returned in the One-Step which superseded the popularity of the Two-Step as the second favourite to the Waltz during the first decade of the new century. The One-Step had already been visible as an occasional version of the Two-Step (see Humphrey, 1911a, 1911c). It was quite simply a rhythmic walk, the weight being transferred from foot to foot as the dancers moved around the room. It could as easily be danced to a 6/8 as to a 2/4. But it was the syncopated character of the ragtime music that gave the dance its driving force and character. Dancers tended to accentuate the musical rhythm by jerkily moving their outstretched arms up and down. This pumping action was often accompanied by moving shoulders and swaying hips. Furthermore, the dance's simplicity encouraged dancers to vary their progress around the room by taking differently sized steps and sudden moves into new directions, as the mood took them. The liveliness of syncopation and the new brasher instrumentation of ragtime bands particularly appealed to the young, as did the fact that the dancing could be imitated almost immediately. Expensive and time consuming lessons with a dancing master were no longer counted essential in order to 'rag' a dance.

There were numerous variations on the One-Step emanating from the United States, first the Judy Walk and later the infamous Turkey Trot, the most prominent of a succession of so-called animal dances such as the Grizzly Bear and the Bunny Hug. New dances were hailed by exhibition dancers, theatrical entrepreneurs and the press alike, as the latest phenomenon poised to hit the fashionable dancing scene.[4] The shock value of a new invention, as the successful careers of musical theatre stars and exhibition dancers suggested, afforded ready cultural capital, however ridiculous the dancing might appear to those of more conservative tastes. A route to upward social mobility might lie, *Punch* playfully advised, in the creation of 'a sillier and more undignified dance than has ever been danced before'.[5]

The press lampooned the seeming flood of new ragtime dances by citing fictitious examples: the Puppy Hug, the Chicken Crawl, the Milwaukee Move Along-Please, and the Monkey Scramble.[6] The associations with animals often 'from the farmyard', the foregrounding of movements not normally associated with dancing but with indecorous social behaviour, and the suggestion of origins in African-American territory in these titles were characteristic of the new dances. More significantly, they pointed to what was perceived as a trilogy of worrying trends in society: animalistic behaviour, the decline of civilization, and the foreignness of popular culture, especially African-American music and dance. In general, the more novel ragtime concoctions, even if based upon actual African-American popular social dancing, made a comparatively limited appearance on the English dance floor. Knowledge of the more extreme moves such as lifts, bending very far backwards, or squatting was acquired chiefly from watching theatrical performances or reading sensationalist press accounts.[7]

Tango-mania

In Paris during the opening years of the twentieth century, the Tango had a small but dedicated following among rich Argentinean émigrés and in the café culture of Montmartre (see Cooper in Collier et al., 1995; Savigliano, 1995). Following his realization that the Tango's existing manifestation was unsuitable for polite society, Camille De Rhynal, with other enthusiasts, including the Grand Duchess Anastasia of Russia, began to re-work the dance at the Imperial Country Club in Nice before later promoting it through dedicated competitions in Paris (Silvester and Richardson, 1936). Embraced by Parisian high society and performed by music-hall stars Mistinguett and Max Dearly, the Tango, now performed to a more romantic habanera rhythm, became the next dance craze to sweep across Europe and North America. Belle Harding learned the dance in 1911, at De Rhynal's Parisian studio which though 'like an old barn' attracted 'a wonderful collection of carriages belonging to the most notable people of the French capital' (Harding quoted in Silvester and Richardson, 1936, p. 29). From here, the neophyte dancers went on to *thés dansants* run by De Rhynal in the Palais Persan at the Magic City dance hall near to the Eiffel Tower. For British devotees of the Tango, interest peaked in the winter dancing season following the dance's huge success with holiday makers returning in the autumn of 1912 from the northern French Riviera (see Figure 15.1).[8]

Unlike ragtime dances, the Tango required considerable knowledge and skill to participate on the dance floor, and its arrival was greeted by high levels of popular demand for tuition and by opportunistic invention of associated commodities. Tango music, Tango dresses, Tango corsets, even a special colour, a bright shade of orange, were branded and marketed as Tango essentials. London socialite Gladys Beattie Crozier (1913) published a whole book dedicated to the dance, lifting without acknowledgement much of *The Dancing Times*'s guide to the best dancing venues in London. She advised the Tango-hungry public where to go to enjoy the dance and provided scantily researched information on the dance's history, music, dress, and choreography. Copiously illustrated with photographs of exhibition dancers Los Almanos from Paris demonstrating their latest figures, Crozier's book also offered advice on how to organize a tango tea and, included a chapter on another fashion – how to perform the Tango on roller skates.[9]

In contrast to the expansive Boston, the non-progressive Argentine Tango was ideally suited to the restricted spaces of drawing rooms and restaurants. In the years immediately prior to the First World War,

164

THE LATEST FASHION : "Pour Passer le Temps."

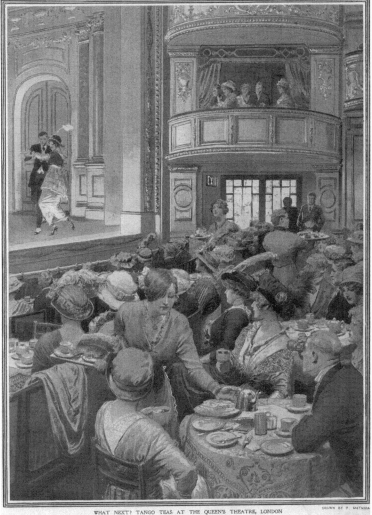

WHAT NEXT? TANGO TEAS AT THE QUEEN'S THEATRE, LONDON

DRAWN BY F. MATANIA

The novelty of the hour is the tango tea. It may be seen at the Queen's Theatre, London, with the stalls removed and replaced by tables and chairs for afternoon tea. The band is on the stage, where M. Clayton and Mlle. Marquis give us tango dances, and this is supplemented by a down pursuit of all the latest fashions

Figure 15.1   The Latest Fashion: "Pour Passer le Temps", *The Sphere*, 11 October 1913

the Parisian innovation of dinner dances had been introduced, couples moving onto the dance floor between courses to dance. It was not until 1913 that dance clubs were opened in London for the express purpose of dancing. Most notable among these were the 400 Club in Old Bond Street, later to become the Embassy Club, the Lotus Club (Garrick Street), Ciro's Club (Orange Street), and Murray's Club in Beak Street.[10] Unlike the afternoon *thés dansants*, these were supper clubs where the rich, fashionable and decadent could dance the night away.

Noted for its close body contact, sinuous grace, and potential erotic allure, the Tango initially gained ground among the dedicated dance enclaves of the London upper-middle class. By 1911, it was already popular at the subscription dances of the Royalist Club but enjoyed widespread fame in Britain in response to its much hyped rendition by musical theatre performers Phyllis Dare and George Grossmith Junior in the 1912 Gaiety production, *The Sunshine Girl*. Grossmith Junior received instruction in the Argentine Tango from Parisian salon hostess Madame Jean de Reske (Richardson, 1946; Silvester and Richardson, 1936), though the photographic series of dramatic poses in *The Sketch*, cigarette in hand and rose in mouth, elucidate the dance's transformation from a social form to one designed for exotic theatrical appeal. Such imagery and countless performances, either directly imitative of Dare and Grossmith or culled from numerous other theatrical sources, were milked by the press to feed the public appetite for Tango.[11]

A regular press item, the Tango was given undue and erroneous prominence as a salacious dance, condemned by the Queen of England and the Pope. The former had actually exercised no such judgement, although it was true that none of the recently imported dances figured on the court ball programme. The press rumour was scotched when Maurice Mouvet and Florence Walton were invited to perform the Tango in the royal presence at a garden party in 1914.[12] By then, the Tango had run its course as the supposed *bête noire* of the establishment, and leisure venue proprietors, dancing teachers, and the press had already begun to look for the next dance craze in the Brazilian Maxixe, the Furlana, the Tao Tao, and the Foxtrot. The Tango had also become overly complicated for the average dancer. It had initially been considered too difficult with its myriad figures and the choreographic demands made upon the male dancer to initiate the selection of material while on the dance floor. Just as the Boston had diversified into named variants when dancing teachers aimed to meet clientele interest for greater novelty, the figures of the Argentine Tango became subject to such invention that there arose innumerable steps and figures to be learned. Tango dancers attending events without their familiar partners or wishing to meet new partners could find themselves at a loss when trying to match their knowledge on the dance floor. The Tango vogue had burnt out by early 1914 in fashionable society, though among dedicated dancers, it occasionally appeared in London and would significantly re-emerge from Paris in the post-war years in a new, progressive form.

In the final dancing season before hostilities broke out, the number of fresh initiatives gave Richardson cause to comment on the year's significance for Britain's dance culture, pointing to the introduction of tango teas, the rapid increase in the number of exhibition ballroom dancers, and the appearance of supper dances at the élite West End clubs where dancing could be enjoyed late into the night.[13] The war might have halted the progressive speed and spread of such developments, but their contribution to the visibility and public character of dancing would be foundational for the patterns of kinetic expression that greeted the return of peacetime.

Dancing through the war years

The declaration of war in August 1914 forced many British tourists and workers, including dance instructors such as Mme Vandyck who was teaching in fashionable Baden Baden, to beat a hasty retreat from the continent.[14] Even if London visitors were prepared for the extra five hours of travel to Paris on the only direct route between Folkestone and Dieppe by late 1914, the capital of night-time hedonistic culture was veiled under curfew after eight o'clock in the evening.[15] In Britain, the government had hastily implemented the Defence of the Realm Act (DORA) which included among its myriad prohibitions (added to as the war progressed) restrictions on the consumption of alcohol, gas, electricity, coal, and food. Adult dancing classes fell away as the nation committed itself to the war effort, the consequential impact on the income of many older dancing teachers resulting in the coffers of pedagogic associations being called upon to assist members in distress. The first experiences of Zeppelin air raids in 1915 were an additional reason to limit evening public entertainment. Such seemingly frivolous pursuits as dancing initially appeared unpatriotic, as a generation of young men volunteered to go to the front. It later became clear, however, that dancing proved excellent relaxation for soldiers on leave, anxious to meet up with relatives and friends and to enjoy female company in an atmosphere where they might forget the horrors of war. There were some proprietors and clientele, mostly at private nightclubs, who transgressed the limited freedoms of entertainment which, as war deepened, resulted in a ban on officers appearing at dances in uniform. In the closing months of the war, however, largely consequent upon the arrival of American allies, such restrictions were lifted, leading to renewed charity dances mounted with the approval of the military authorities.[16]

While producing a much reduced *Dancing Times*, published in line with austerity measures, its editor, too old for fighting, contributed to the war effort as a special constable in London. Recognizing the need to build morale and a future foundation for dance activity when the war was over, through the pages of his journal, Richardson advocated a national approach to improving dance training and pedagogy and expanded the monthly column, 'Gossip from the States'. In part, this latter feature was a consequence of the moratorium on reports from special correspondents on the continent, but direct communication across the Atlantic grew apace.

Dominant dances during the war were the One-Step, the Hesitation Waltz – a variant on the Waltz which introduced a rhythmic pause – and increasingly a new dance, the Foxtrot which made its entrance in London just before the outbreak of war. Richardson initially thought its chances of success within the British social dance repertoire were limited. Indeed, when Stroud Haxton's band at the 400 Club first played Foxtrot music in July 1914, the dancers, Richardson among them, were puzzled as to how to respond (Silvester and Richardson, 1936). The dance was soon promoted on the stage, especially in musical comedies and revues, such as *To-night's the Night* at the Gaiety, *5064 Gerrard* at the Alhambra and notably in the song 'Show Us How to Do the Fox-trot' featured at the Empire in *Watch Your Step*, the first full-time ragtime musical from Irving Berlin which had proved so successful a vehicle for the dancing talents of the Castles, their roles in Britain being undertaken by American actors and singers Ethel Levey and Joseph Coyne.[17] Edinburgh teacher D. G. MacLennan, resident in London during the war years, was one of the first to demonstrate the Foxtrot to the profession, having already encountered the Foxtrot when teaching on summer schools for the American Dancing Masters Association in the summer of 1914. Belle Harding, ever at the forefront of new initiatives, also championed the dance through classes and competition.[18]

The Foxtrot was in a very fluid condition when it first arrived, best described at the time as a 'go-as-you-please' dance, its most distinguishing feature being a sequence of slow and quick steps. The simplest variant was four slow steps (each taking two beats) followed by seven quick steps and a pause before recommencing. Existing dances were drawn upon by participants on the floor to provide choreographic content, although a myriad new steps and figures such as respectively a 'twinkle' and 'butterfly' appeared. In character, the Foxtrot was far removed from the smooth, gliding dance known to the later twentieth century. Josephine Bradley recalled being 'borne away with "perky" walks, trotting runs, and perhaps, thrill of thrills, a jaunty twinkle',[19] in 1917, although the Saunter, a more leisurely form that required greater technical control to achieve smooth transference of weight, championed by *The Dancing Times* in 1916, was ultimately to have a *rallentando* effect on the Foxtrot.[20] For the time though, the two forms, the jaunty Foxtrot and more dreamy Saunter co-existed, before further war restrictions on leisure during 1917 deadened any chance of further developments in the ballroom.

Towards the end of that year, however, on the United States' entry into the war, the radical new sound of jazz re-energized the fashionable dance floors of London. As American soldiers galvanized the dance scene bringing new bands from across the Atlantic, there was confusion in Britain over the meaning of 'jazz' (Parsonage, 2005). Attempting to fit the name to previous trends, for a while, it was erroneously thought by many that the term represented a new dance or at least a new step.

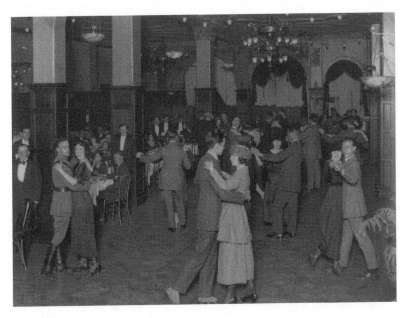

Figure 15.2   Ballroom Dancing, Murray's Club

Indeed, for a while, a combination consisting of three steps to four counts of music was termed a jazz roll, first making its appearance according to Richardson at Murray's Club (Silvester and Richardson, 1936), a venue then popular with the American troops. The combination was later to emerge as the 'three-step' in the Foxtrot, though in the labile dance situation of the time, exponents were as likely to introduce it into any other dance (see Figure 15.2).

Given the lack of opportunity for regular practice and tuition in war time, the 'go-as-you-please' nature of the One-Step and Foxtrot gained ascendancy in the ballroom. The involvement of often older relatives on the dance floor, familiar with the Waltz from earlier years, contributed to the retention of affection for the European dance rhythm; new dancers, though, struggled to revolve fully and smoothly. In the years following the war, the Waltz was to rise from the ashes; but that it did so, along with other social dances, owed much to the concerted efforts of professional dancers, pedagogues, the press, and dedicated amateur dancers, aiming to restore civilization to a land anxious to recover from the threats of invasion, both physical and cultural.

16
Knuts and Aliens

[N]ever surely was there so much terpsichorean activity as in the years immediately preceding the outbreak
of the Great War.

Ralph Nevill, *Echoes Old and New*, 1919, p. 303

Changing social relations between young men and women had been
clearly visible in the ballroom from the early 1900s; the reluctant masher
and sad figure of the wallflower of the 1890s had passed into memory,
being replaced by the keen dancing man of fashion known as a 'knut' or
'nut' and the fun-loving more independent young woman of the 1910s.[1]
No longer courtly and restrained, the fashionable dancing of the early
1900s epitomized the new craving for freedom from former constraints
in social interaction and modes of corporeality. Desire and aspiration to
be modish propelled those with free time, spending power and the right
social contacts towards a lifestyle of fashionable consumerism, marked
as young, energetic, cosmopolitan, urbane, and expensive. Fresh models of gendered deportment and dress arose which embodied emphasis
upon self-expression, mobility, and rapid transformation.

Knuts and modern girls in the ballroom

Bon viveur and author Ralph Nevill (1919, p. 300), reflecting upon male
pleasures just after the First World War, recalled that by 1913 a new type
of man-about-town had emerged who was distinctive in his 'dress, habits, mode of thought and mode of life'. Unlike the previous generation's
young bloods, mashers and dandies who had enjoyed the night pleasures of drink, women, gambling, and fighting, the new man-about-town
appeared altogether more sophisticated, interested in art, the opera and

170

theatre, as well as enjoying the costly leisure pursuits of motoring and golf. The 'more frivolous' among these, Nevill (1919, p. 301) observed, possessed 'a perfect mania for dancing'. Whereas, the earlier masher and conventional late-Victorian young man had been imprisoned in starched collars and waistcoats, male dress was now becoming more relaxed. For the ultra-fashionable male, termed the 'Super Nut' by Crozier, the tango tea afforded him opportunity to wear 'shining white spats, and even white-topped boots' (1913, p. 128), the less formal morning coat in town (though even the informality of a jacket was acceptable elsewhere) and, the more comfortable half-inch neck collar, while the once *de rigueur* convention of white gloves had been abandoned.[2]

At some Society private dances in the pre-War years, men now reportedly outnumbered the girls.[3] Sceptics murmured that the root cause of sudden male interest in dancing resulted more from the potential for close bodily contact rather than from any genuine terpsichorean passion. Certainly, drawing rooms witnessed an intimate embrace between dancing partners that was once only permissible among the urban working classes and in nightclubs of ill repute. No doubt, some men did take advantage of loosened choreographic parameters, manoeuvring their partners around the floor through close frontal body contact, rather than by the more subtle and socially approved signals from the man's hand on his partner's upper back and outstretched hand to guide her. The distance between partners espoused by high-class Victorian dancing masters for couple dancing now impeded quick and easy responses by female partners in the new improvisational repertoire. In any case, a more relaxed stance and closer contact was gaining acceptance, even if the conservative *Punch* typically exaggerated the situation for satirical effect (see Figure 16.1).

If the new music and dances lured men back into the ballroom through the attraction of exciting new rhythms and close physical contact with the opposite sex: the Boston[4] and, more especially, the Tango, played an important part through offering the prospect of demonstrating individual skill on the dance floor. In spite of the notorious emotional reserve of the British middle and upper classes, the capacity to improvise also chimed with notions of manliness. As an amateur dancer and Fleet Street journalist observed:

> The tango is an ideal dance for the man. He creates the design of it throughout, and in doing this calls into play mental as well as physical prowess, and as he develops a mastery over many divers steps the more elaborate and interesting to him becomes the designing of the

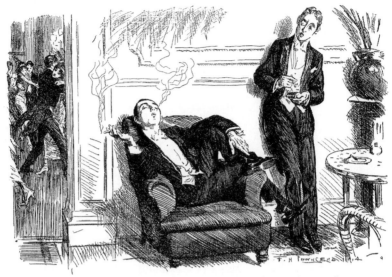

Reclining Nut. "I don't bother to hold the girls now-a-days, I just let 'em nestle."

Figure 16.1   Reclining Nut, *Punch*, 18 March 1914

dance. He has no uncomfortably close or tight hold of the lady, yet his control of the lady's movements is more complete than in the waltz.[5]

The Tango reinforced gender norms of male leadership, and, like the earlier Waltz, celebrated the heterosexual couple. Now 'free from all erotic taint', it provided an excellent vehicle for the British dancer to showcase culturally approved masculine traits.[6] Furthermore, the dance afforded the man a chance to exercise his individuality 'that supremely male and Victorian ideology' (Duffin, 1978, p. 74) which now found kinetic expression in the early twentieth-century ballroom.

The dance floor provided new freedoms of heterosexual bodily contact not to be indulged in public elsewhere. Chaperones were rarely to be seen and limitations on the number of dances a Society girl might promise to one partner fell away as female emancipation gathered pace.[7] It was observed that no modern woman arrived at a dance without a partner and indeed often came with several. In a remarkable reversal, any individual left to sit out a dance was now more than likely to be male. In any case, the complexities of the Tango and its numerous variations favoured the retention of one previously known partner throughout the event, an exigency which ran counter to the Victorian dream of the ballroom as a Utopian microcosm of society, drawing all, young and old, into the fold. The Society ballroom increasingly became the province of the young, and young at heart, their modern music rejected by many among the older generation as alien, uncivilized, and unmelodic, its accompanying movement as barbaric, immoral and ugly. Youth became synonymous with modernity, open and eager for new experiences.[8]

As political and social ascendancy moved away from the British aristocracy with a consequential demise in the matriarchal power of Society wives, a new ideal of femininity had emerged: single, slim, healthy, physically active and, most of all, youthful. The Gaiety Girls had been influential as new ideals of female beauty, perhaps best signalled by the succession of musical comedies with the word 'girl' in the title. From 1908, dress fashions for women accentuated this youthful ideal, regardless of the biological age of their clients. Diaphanous evening wear was designed to cling to a slim figure supported by lighter corsetry, thus allowing for greater freedom of movement. Paradoxically the hobble skirt of 1911 prevented such kinetic emancipation, causing the *Birmingham Despatch* to conjecture wryly that tight ballroom gowns, the limbs often shackled below the knee, were surely responsible for the frequency of the Two-Step on contemporary dance programmes.[9] The appearance of the Tango, however, had a more fortuitous impact upon female liberty with respect to ease of movement and dress. The slit skirts of so-called Tango dresses, the skirt line usually cut two inches above the ground, facilitated the performance of long steps and an occasional 'dip' (though such moves were frowned on in the more staid ballrooms). Society decorum might be observed by wearing the Orientalist-inspired adaptations of Turkish trousers known as harem skirts (though these were never so popular in London as in Paris) or, more usually, by 'chiffon under-draperies' available in the designs of high class fashion houses (Crozier, 1913, p. 123). The shorter split skirts also featured the neat, usually black high-heeled shoes, kept strapped on by cross gartered ribbons or elastic and perfect for pivoting on easily in response to the man's improvisational manoeuvring. A further impact on fashion occasioned by the Tango was the acceleration in decline of the very wide-brimmed hats earlier made popular by *The Merry Widow* (and hated by theatre-goers unable to view the stage) in favour of neat small hats, ideal for dancers adapting to the Tango's more intimate body hold and on the crowded floors at afternoon *thés dansants*.

The styling of Parisian-based Paul Poiret and London aristocratic London designer Lucile (Lady Duff Gordon) fostered a distinctive fashionable pose and mode of moving for women, humorously illustrated by a *Punch*

cartoon which depicts couples at a smart garden party.[10] Observing a bolt upright young woman stylishly dressed, a male guest ponders why she looks 'all wrong somehow' in spite of her prettiness and fashionable attire. His female companion waspishly agrees: 'The ridiculous woman persists in wearing her backbone, and backbones are quite gone out.' Indeed, the new fashion of curved spines, rounded shoulders and the manner of draping both fabric and body lines celebrated the antithesis of Victorian corporeal ideals.

Arguments for, though mostly against, the 'scandalous travesties of dancing' raged back and forth across the national quality press, and were echoed across Society journals, local newspapers, from church pulpits and at dinner tables up and down the country. The chorus of disapproval, mostly from the more elderly and conservative, from senior members of Society and from established teachers of dancing reached a crescendo in summer 1913 in the debate sparked by a letter to *The Times* signed by 'A Peeress.'[11] The anonymous peeress protested that hostesses in the London Season should advise ball-goers in advance if such dances were to feature; an indication on the invitation card, she suggested, might alert the aristocratic matron to avoid such houses so that she might protect her young 'well-brought up girl'. This combination of allusions to the potential contravention of sexual propriety, the glamour and misdemeanours of aristocracy and prurient fascination with the shock of risqué novelties no doubt helped to boost publication sales. Marketing issues aside, however, the high level of attention paid to the topic underlined the socio-cultural importance then attached to dancing and expressed genuine concerns, as well as enthusiasm in some quarters, for what was widely regarded as rupture with the past.

Antagonism towards the new repertoire was by no means peculiar to Britain, but blazed across Eurocentric enclaves as opinion divided. Typically, moral panic was voiced as a concern for the well-being of the impressionable young who were keen to learn the fashionable dances. Numerous, yet often interlinked, accusations were levelled at the new repertoire. It was judged to be barbaric, vulgar, anti-social, immoral, lacking in technique, ugly, low class, animalistic, alien, and decidedly un-English: such epithets centred on the concept of civilization, the maintenance of which, constructed as a peculiarly English phenomenon, was charged by many social commentators to be under threat.

Devotees of the new dancing, however, rejected the repertoire of their parents and grandparents as 'cold, set, pompous dances. ... irksome and uninspiring', incapable of fulfilling contemporary desire for 'individual taste and enterprise'.[12] It is clear that what enthusiasts relished about the new repertoire of dances was the freedom to improvise, to move as the music urged them, regardless of appearance to the onlooker. Self-expression, now a guiding mantra for the lifestyle of the young and rich, had become elevated on the dance floor to an artistic dictate.

It was viewed otherwise by the likes of Edward Scott who condemned the modern dancers who 'rush helter-skelter about a ballroom, darting hither and thither, without any regard to their own appearance or the comfort of other people'.[13] The once decorous dancing in the ballroom now looked, moaned the ISDT's *Dance Journal*, like a 'whirling, jumbled pantomime' in which dancers made 'either a mad rush, or ... [a] studious endeavour to avoid collisions'. Even the less censorious *Dancing Times* complained of the couple who suddenly moved 'like a tongue of flame' across the dance floor.[14]

Staunch advocates of the old round style of dancing expressed doubt that unchecked investment in spontaneity, individuality, and originality were necessarily intentional choreographic choices. Professions of originality, in their view, often belied terpsichorean incompetence, demonstrated a lack of consideration for others and clearly resulted in the loss of personal decorum. *Punch* agreed, gleefully recognizing an old target on the modern dance floor – the bad dancer – and coupled satirical criticism of kinetic ineptitude, epitomized in the figure of 'The Sleuth Stalker'[15] along with the magazine's long-established objective of mocking the gullibility of followers of fashion. 'How much longer', *Punch* asked in 1912,

> are our daughters and sisters to be trundled about like wardrobes, their arms worked incessantly like the parish pump, made to slide about sideways like ungainly crustaceans, and submitted to "Bunny Hugs" and other exotic abominations, which made them look as supremely foolish and vulgar as they can be made to look?[16]

Further public attention to the 'exotic' origins of the dances was to yield deep-seated prejudices that initially, under the guise of aesthetic disapproval, characteristically entwined social, moral, and racial dimensions into the chorus of disapproval and alarm. Earlier discontent with events on the dance floor during the 1890s had hailed the onset of degeneration. What was distinctive in the diatribe during the early 1910s against 'uncivilized' dancing was the focus upon race. In critics' eyes, these later successful attempts to enliven the ballroom, through the introduction of the 'exotica' of 'Half American, half Spanish' couple dances had ousted the naturalized British repertoire of a largely central European-sourced collection of dances. The threats posed to the British dance floor now came not primarily from within the country, but, more worryingly, from outside the European continent, from a new nation of mixed cultural and racial origins: not just America, but more specifically, black America. For, as a *Times* article observed:

> [T]he naive enjoyment of noise and capering as ends in themselves which marks many departments of American life ... has borrowed many of its saltatory expressions from the revels of the Negro population.[17]

Terpsichorean provenance and racial degeneration

The adoption of music and dance forms and practices that were both American and sourced from African and Hispanic cultures was perceived by critics to endanger British culture just at a time when accepted certainties of social status, gender, occupation, money, and power were in considerable flux. The sheer rapidity of change was unsettling to many of more privileged means. Widespread strikes, the growing trades union movement, reforms to the British political constitution to empower the workers, the public disorder of the Suffragette movement, the need for aristocrats to find employment beyond their estates, the continuing rise of the *nouveaux riches*, and the slow decline of the British Empire as the world's premier power had contributed to a sense of unease among Society, as well as among the more conservative upper- and lower-middle classes, for whom the gentility of civilization was compatible with the notion that 'God is an Englishman'. For its white subjects, the civilization of the Britons (for which read English) represented the highest human achievement; the rapid adoption of cultural practices from people who occupied a lower status both within and outside the empire was thus a source of public concern.

British critical response to the new repertoire certainly shared much in common with the moral panic evident in white America.[18] Issues of race, gender, class, and religion appear in the reactions to the new style of dancing on both sides of the Atlantic, complainants often employing similar vocabulary and turns of phrase. Differing socio-historical and cultural circumstances in the two countries, however, resulted in local inflections. Whereas white inhabitants of urban America, especially Chicago, San Francisco, and New York, might take advantage of geographical proximity to witness African-American social dancing, the British experience, in general, was much more distanced.[19] In contrast to America, where large numbers of black people were resident as a result of the Atlantic slave trade, Britain's black population during the decades before the First World War was 'miniscule and fragmented' (Walvin, 1973, p. 202). Writing on entertainment in the London music halls of the period, Horace Barnes (1908, p. 744) declared that 'there is practically no race prejudice in England' though the offensive public commentary less than four years later on the popularity of ragtime music and its performers blatantly contradicted such a naïve and ignorant assertion.

Knowledge of black people in late Victorian and Edwardian Britain primarily depended upon centuries of gross caricatures, recycled and expanded upon in travel literature, cartoons, and theatrical representations. Intransigent opinion on the inferiority of all non-white peoples was endemic in late Victorian and Edwardian British culture.[20] On both sides of the Atlantic, black people were imagined and treated as if stupid, greedy, lazy, deceitful, and promiscuous, incapable of creating and sustaining art, technology, and moral attributes that signalled, through a Eurocentric lens, the state of civilization. The ideology of social Darwinism placed people of African origin at the bottom of the evolutionary tree, biologically close to animals and in their emotional, intellectual and moral development in a permanent state of child-like simplicity. Such a supposed condition legitimated colonialist rule by their 'superiors'.

The biological concept of race, supported by the majority of Victorian scientists, philosophers, and thinkers of note served to 'explain' the comparative economic and cultural power of nations. In this racist and hierarchical vision of humanity, the English positioned themselves as unquestionably born to rule over the world. Their sense of superiority ranged across the full gamut of prejudice: from blatant and damaging racism towards people of differently coloured skin, to a xenophobic attitude towards those of Caucasian appearance, but who were born outside England, Scotland, and Wales and therefore could not be classed as rising from British stock. Prejudice against the so-called Latin races, loosely grouping Spanish, Portuguese, Italian, and French together, emphasized attributed traits of excessive sensitivity, sensuality, laziness, lack of courage, and an inability to control feelings, especially those of a sexual nature. Such ascribed traits, overlapping with many that were already believed to be typical of black people, followed deeply held normative values of whiteness (Dyer, 1997).

Alien bodily actions

Commentators on the transatlantic source of the new repertoire recognized the dances' popularity as but one aspect of the growing cultural hegemony of the United States, whether through 'subtle permeation of our way of life by the American sense of the dignity of bustle' or, 'continuously forcing [their] way ... with the peculiar persistence of all things American'.[21] The conviction that all Americans, regardless of colour, were culturally backward with a 'poor conception of the poetry of motion' remained strong in British thought, though it was sometimes countered by English dancers with experience of the European elite-derived dance culture of the more prosperous white Americans.[22] The latest dances from the New World, however, were regarded in many traditionalist quarters as a disconcerting breach with traditional European aesthetics and manners.

The establishment's sense of affront and distaste for ragtime is emphatically distilled in cartoon form by artist and imperialist Leonard Raven-Hill (see Figure 16.2).[23] The Hellenic personification of civilized Music stops her ears in alarm, Terpsichore's lyre dropped behind her, as out from a box labelled 'A Present from USA' spring American entertainers, arms and legs jutting at angles, hands splayed, like so many disjointed puppets, as they bawl out musical comedy numbers. The caption, 'Time, Gentlemen, Please!' plays on the sense of ragtime as broken time or suggests an inability of the musicians to keep time. It further references the publican's habitual order to drink up and go home and, by extension, the growing association by critics of ragtime with its enthusiasts' perceived loss of control. The feared threat to civilization could not be more graphically illustrated: the old versus the new, the elite versus the popular and Hellenic cultural origins versus sources in Africa.

In the attacks on the new repertoire, two familiar conservative and bourgeois targets were lined up for the shots of moral disapproval: the theatre, especially in its popular guise, and members of the aristocracy, bent on seeking novel pleasures.[24] On the stage, complainants argued, American and continental performers were demonstrating dance moves that were quite unacceptable in a civilized ballroom. Prurient hypocrisy, however, was clearly abroad: 'the more daring the dance, the more it is appreciated and applauded by the very same individuals who would be horrified at the performance of a mild "Bunny Hug" in their own drawing-rooms' noted one correspondent.[25] Indeed, complained Cecil Taylor, president of the ISDT, the chief offenders in courting and supporting the new repertoire were the very people, those 'moving in the highest circles', that should be setting examples as models of decorum.[26] It was the male 'younger bloods' of aristocracy who early in the summer of 1910 had reputedly opened up the doors of wealthy Mayfair to the Bohemian, mainly young female, cast of theatreland with whom they were already socially familiar. In the early hours of a spring morning, at

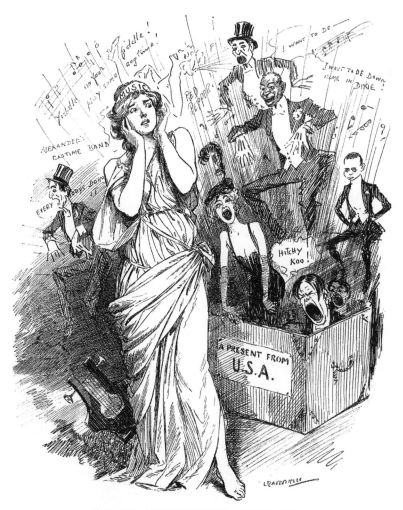

"TIME, GENTLEMEN, PLEASE!"

Figure 16.2   Time, Gentlemen, Please, *Punch*, 9 April 1913

the Grafton Galleries, all convention was swept aside as they ate, drank, sang, indulged in horse-play, and danced 'to the music of a darkey band, which played rag-time almost too emotionally'.[27]

Such enthusiasm for the new music was damned by Edward Scott who condemned its propensity to stimulate movements, even in high-class hotel ballrooms, that in his eyes were, at best, little more than 'wriggling

to music'. Through his many lecture-demonstrations and prolific publication, Scott relentlessly alerted public attention to ragtime's African sources
and conducted a prominent and vicious campaign against a 'style of dancing that might be tolerated, or even admired, among semi-barbarous races'
but which 'becomes vulgar and disgusting when exhibited in an English
ball-room'.[28] He remained adamant that it was the teacher's expert duty to
exorcise those dances from the repertoire in which 'alien bodily actions'
were present in order to 'keep our dancing pure.'[29]

Any hint of poor taste (a euphemism for sexual expression) on the
dance floor, however, was held by many critics of the new dancing to
be a characteristic of other races. 'One or two couples, the gentleman
are foreigners ... add to great natural grace an unnecessary touch of
the amorous in their movements' wrote one chaperone.[30] Latin male
dancers, such as Brazilian Senor Marquis and Argentine Almanos, now
appeared in smart European venues as high-profile demonstrators, teachers, and partners of the Tango and Maxixe. Often their female partners
were not Latina, fuelling the popular image of the Latin as a gigolo,
paid by women for more than his dancing services. Small wonder that
Victorian dancing masters D'Egville and Scott hated the Tango; to them,
the dance epitomized the complete opposite of the ideal British male.
Only in the Anglo-Saxon Menuet de la Cour and the Waltz might manliness and chivalry be personified; never in the Latin Tango and Maxixe.[31]
These dances in Scott's eyes were marked with exhibitionist sensuality
and effeminacy, evidence of degeneration towards a less civilized state
(Chamberlin and Gilman, 1985). The man's role was to provide for and
to protect women, not to indulge in exhibitions of imitative sex on the
dance floor: certainly, Scott proclaimed, he was no gentleman who
moved his hips when dancing.

Rejecting press warnings of moral degeneration and alternative dance
repertoires from the old English court and countryside, most amateur
dancers took up the continental and transatlantic novelties. The pur-
ported barbarism of the new dances was, by no means, interpreted as
the end of civilization, but rather the potential for a new, more genuine
beginning in creative self-expression. Personal artistic enunciation was
a leitmotif of the period and, if inspiration was no longer to be found in
European civilization, then it might legitimately be drawn from so-called
primitive culture where rule had not yet deadened instinct and creativity. George Grossmith Junior defended the new dances by articulating
the popular belief in a supposed natural affinity of black people for
movement and rhythm. Was the alleged origin of the dances in African
culture, he argued 'wholly a reproach where dancing is concerned?' (in

Naylor, 1913, p. 226). Positioned as further from artifice and closer to
nature, this new kinetic material, evoking the long-repressed frisson
of primitive sexuality, however remote and attributed, held out the
sought-after cachet of authentic origins in the exotic (erotic) Other.

For keen social dancers, however, corporeal contact with the opposite
sex was but one attraction of the new repertoire. More important was
the opportunity 'just to dream with their music and be seized with the
spirit of volition' (Hyatt-Woolf, 1911, p. 5). Improvisation was hailed as
spontaneous, free from meaningless convention, natural, without artifice and correspondingly authentic. Indeed, wrote the same enthusiast,
'the dancing of the moment is very akin to Post-impressionism, or rather
what their devotees claim for it – an expression of the emotions, the real
ecstasy of the spirit of the music' (Hyatt-Woolf, 1911, p. 5). It is not then
without significance that when the revellers of Bohemia and Mayfair met
in 1910 to dance ragtime, the walls of the Grafton Galleries were hung
with Manet's pictures. For the dancers, modernity was equated with corporeal freedom, the music lending wings to the 'spirit of revolt and desire
of escape' to fly to a happy place where 'for a little while the emotions
may be unfettered ... where one's real nature ... may ring free.'[32] Such
individualism and championing of the loss of self-consciousness flew
in the face of all the expertise and values of Society Victorian dancing
teachers and their followers.

17
Civilizing from the Centre

> I always think that the best dancers in the room are
> the couples you notice last of all.
> Anti-Standardization, *The Dancing Times*,
> January 1918, p. 128

The new century saw further dance-teacher associations formed along-side and often in competition with the BATD and the ISDT (re-named the Imperial Society of Teachers of Dancing in 1925). These included the United Kingdom Alliance of Professional Teachers of Dancing established in 1903 in Manchester which included social dance, operatic dancing and sword fencing within its remit, and the National Association of Teachers of Dancing which began life early in 1907 in South London as the Southern Association of Teachers of Dancing.[1] The professed aim of all was to agree standardization of dances, to provide financial (and sometimes legal) support for its members in times of distress, to disseminate new dances, and to elevate the art of dancing to the highest standards. Some associations, like the ISDT, were outward-facing, sending delegates to international conferences of dance teachers in Paris. Favoured by Richardson as the organization most capable of effecting improvement and unity in the pedagogic profession, the ISDT took the lead, under Richardson's direction, of proposing and formulating agreed syllabuses for the teaching of modern ballroom dancing in the 1920s.[2]

The other associations, featuring fewer luminaries among their teachers than the ISDT, focused more on the needs of their lower-middle class clientele. Reluctant to adopt the repertoire of the West End, the instructors concentrated instead on the composition of new sequence dances, easily learned and capable of variation within the constraints of the old

Victorian technique. Richardson was initially snobbish in his attitude towards these teachers and their associations. His new magazine was angled towards the higher end of the market of dance enthusiasts and professionals. He was astute, however, in identifying dance trends and expanding his readership. By 1912, his magazine included reports from the teachers' associations, as well as a popular monthly item 'Round the Classes', accompanied by photographs of pupils from schools up and down the country. The item was mutually promotional for the editor and the teachers, but the esteemed veteran teacher D'Egville was disparaging about such developments, particularly the advertising of qualifications to teach, which now the associations bestowed upon their qualified members. D'Egville's argument was that a true master of art needed no such legitimation, especially as the examinations set by the associations did not assess teaching ability (D'Egville, 1937).

The royal dancing master's scorn for professional organisations and their attempts to control standards through examinations relate to a bygone age; for younger generations of teachers, professional accreditation was thought essential to their career and to the raising of standards. Richardson was unstinting in his quest to promote quality through institutional means, calling for a central body, a 'Royal College of Dancing'. He saw an opportunity in the national Teachers' Registration Council of 1912 and urged teachers of dancing to make representation to that organization. The Council did not include dancing in its remit, privileging gymnastics and physical exercise instead. In the exchange of letters between the ISDT and the Council, the ISDT put forward its characterization of the qualifications regarded as prerequisites for registration as a qualified dance teacher. These included a minimum age of 25, seven years of teaching experience, a 'sound general education', a minimum of 12 months' instruction in how to teach by a registered teacher, and the possession of a diploma by a recognized society of dance teachers. Richardson's exhortations to all the separate dancing teacher associations and individuals to make a united representation to the Council, however, fell largely on deaf ears: in addition to the lack of an established infrastructure for dance in Britain, there remained rivalries and histories that could not so easily and so quickly be ignored.[3]

By the outbreak of the First World War, the character of dance teaching had shifted considerably towards an increasingly female and middle-class workforce, keen to acquire qualifications from a national professional association, and tending to specialize in either stage or social dancing.[4]

Pre-war strategies of refinement

A formative influence on the modern repertoire was the institution of regular competitions as a means to raise standards and to encourage the adoption of approved holds, steps, and styles. Victorian popular culture had endorsed competition of various kinds, though the traditional pastime of waltzing for prizes was deemed by Society and the imitative bourgeoisie a vulgar pastime of the rural and urban working classes. English ladies of reputation did not put their bodies, even when modestly clothed, on comparative show before the public nor, indeed, did men of social distinction. Towards the century's end, however, competitions to select the best new sequence dance were an annual feature of professional teaching organizations such as the BATD, while at the popular assemblies, in-house competitions for dancers became a regular event. Indeed, Richardson himself later confessed to a youthful second place in a waltzing contest organized by dancing teacher Sidney Bishop.[5]

Over on the continent, however, dance competitions in the early 1900s attracted a mix of professional dancers and aristocrats both as participants and observers. The Cake Walk, not surprisingly, given its pedigree in the United States as a dancing contest (Stearns and Stearns, 1968), was the first imported form to be promoted in a Parisian competition by *Excelsior*, the French capital's popular newspaper.[6] In 1907, Camille De Rhynal organized a Tango Championship Contest in Nice before the World Championships in Tango were held in Paris two years later (Silvester and Richardson, 1936, pp. 27–8). Then, in 1911 Princess Eugène Murat invited *Excelsior* to organize a competition at the Théâtre Femina on the Champs Elysées which attracted a fashionable audience, including not only European aristocrats and royals but also Maurice Mouvet and Mistinguett who were persuaded to give an exhibition.[7]

By this time, private subscription dances in London were following suit by organizing competitions for their own members. Also inspired by the French example, Belle Harding mounted Tango competitions during her summer season at Le Touquet and in 1915 she established the first Foxtrot contests in Britain. Initially, adjudication at these private competitions was primarily by popular vote, but by 1911 the Royalist Club had moved to a committee of judges composed of past winners. This strategy of deploying social dance expertise from the upper-middle classes, as well as expert teachers, rather than relying on populist or theatre celebrity response, was to be strengthened following the war, thus effecting genre specific and genteel criteria of excellence to aid in shaping what would later come to be known as the modern English style of ballroom dancing.[8]

In popular dance historiography, Irene and Vernon Castle have often been afforded the most authoritative position in rendering the ragtime and South American dances suitable for polite ballrooms. Highly paid and well-publicised in their campaign to refine and modernize social dancing, the glamorous couple undoubtedly wielded significant and widespread influence through their performances, social connections, teaching, films, press interviews and publications. They were, though, by no means the first or last to agitate for and effect such changes; the efforts to transform the dances formed part of a transcontinental movement of exhibition dancers, teachers, aristocrats and bourgeoisie working together. As a consequence, perhaps, Richardson found himself 'a trifle disappointed' when their book *Modern Dancing* was published in 1914. Judging it limited in new revelations and lacking clarity in the dance notations, he, nonetheless, reproduced the 'Castle House Suggestions for Correct Dancing', their closing summary of admonitions against the infelicities of contemporary social dancing.

> Do not wriggle the shoulders; do not shake the hips; do not twist the body; do not flounce the elbows; do not pump the arms; do not hop – glide instead; avoid low, fantastic, and acrobatic dips; stand far enough away from each other to allow free movement of the body in order to dance gracefully and comfortably. The gentleman should rest his hand lightly against the lady's back, touching her with the fingertips and wrist only, or, if preferred, with the inside of the wrist and the back of the thumb. The gentleman's left hand and forearm should be held up in the air parallel with his body, with the hand extended, holding the lady's hand lightly on his palm. The arm should never be straightened out. Remember you are at a social gathering, and not in a gymnasium. Drop the Turkey Trot, the Grizzly Bear, the Bunny Hug, etc. These dances are ugly, ungraceful, and out of fashion.[9]

Modernity in the ballroom was all.

Some of the reprehensible dances and moves that were reproduced in the ballroom might have been sourced in the more daring and spectacular dance acts of the music hall and musical comedy, but as American dance historian Danielle Robinson (2010) persuasively argues, the erasure of such elements from polite ballrooms under the rubric of modernization was, in effect, a means of whitening a repertoire that was recognizably African in much of its material. It was also a repertoire that owed much to European traditional couple dance forms and styles of the American urban working class (Robinson, 2009), though these lineages received less overt censure in the racist condemnations of the period. The old enemy had been the vulgarity of the lower orders' dancing, but the very familiarity of the couple dance form, as French dance historian Sophie Jacotot (2007) identifies in relation to the popularity of American dances in France, was a significant factor in their endorsement among white dancers.

In Britain, a more regular and up-to-date strategy for effecting change through publication was, of course, Richardson's *Dancing Times*. In his mid-thirties when he took on its editorship, Richardson forged a singular career in professionalizing and institutionalizing dance, across both social and theatrical realms, in Britain. Visiting the studios of top teachers, interviewing key personnel in the world of dance, attending and reviewing dance in the theatre, as well as participating himself in the better-class subscription dances, Richardson harnessed his knowledge and connections to pull the threatened standard of dancing in Britain upwards through the engine of the magazine and through his well-connected and increasingly authoritative person. His strategies were several: he published articles by respected authorities on dance; carried a regular report on dancing and fashion from Paris and later from New York; encouraged participation in debate through the correspondence columns; employed like-minded writers from his own class of social dancers; elicited opinions by prominent teachers and dancers on issues in the ballroom and ran features on West End fashionable teachers, composers and band leaders. He often ghost wrote articles and notes; attracted advertisers of high-class fashion; initiated occasional competitions to nominate, for example, the best Waltz melody; reviewed the latest and growing number of books on dance; and later acted as competition judge and influential chairman of national and indeed international initiatives in dance. His dedicated aim was to foster and shape a social dance culture that was to be high quality, modern yet civilized and, above all, English. Perhaps most persuasive of all was his lively and topical editorial, positioned prominently and attractively at the front of the magazine, appearing under his habitual *nom de plume* of the 'Sitter Out'.[10] It was predominantly through the postwar *Dancing Times* that the issues of standardization came to a head and through Richardson's strong steer, working in tandem with teachers and dancers, were resolved.

Issues of standardization

The pursuit of individual expression, devoid of skill and consideration for fellow couples on the dance floor, was to evoke, even among the most dedicated respondents to the new music and choreography, a growing recognition of the fact that controls needed to be set. The brake of the First World War, when public dances were periodically under government ban, not only halted developments towards reform and consensus but also added to the problem. Those few men returning from the battlefield were literally out of step with yet further new ways of dancing that were arriving directly from America, rather than via the war-straitened Paris. With the arrival of jazz came yet a further bewildering array of steps. For the increasingly moneyed middle classes, the time had arrived to impose constraints of gentility and order to ensure that the ballroom once again was a safe and pleasurable environment in which to pursue courtship and leisure.

Lacking regular tuition and attending occasional dances on leave in London, where impromptu imitation was often the only resort, young soldiers were at a loss on the dance floor, especially with respect to waltzing which was returning to favour. The influx of jazz and the crowded dance spaces at the end of the war further exacerbated the problems.[11] It was not only the young and inexperienced who needed guidance but also older relatives, keen to enjoy the brief leisure time with loved ones, but schooled in earlier forms of dancing, who did not know how to respond to the new 'nigger bands' and their music. *Punch* as ever captured the bewilderment of the older generation at the myriad and confusing new steps to be learned as a result of jazz. 'It's perfectly simple, Uncle', advises a young child, encouraging him to join the packed dance floor:

> [T]wo slow, three quick, three side chassées, wobble-wobble, lame duck, lame duck, dip, grasshopper, two slow, swivel, scissors, jazz-roll, kick, turn, two chassées, back, twinkle and on again.[12]

The popular press took up the calls to standardize the repertoire to circumvent the chaotic scenes on the floor or the diversity of moves which prevented puzzled neophytes from even stepping onto it. Initially, there was resistance from some dancers. Having won the highly prized facility for self-expression and improvisation on the dance floor, fashionable dancers were loathe to return to the simplicity and potential rowdyism of pre-choreographed dances.[13] But, as so often in Britain, at stake were not merely barriers to kinetic enjoyment, but issues of social status. 'The classes', Richardson advised, meaning the upper-middle classes and above 'insist that their dances shall always bear the hall-mark of Paris or New York before they will take them up'.[14] In contrast, 'the masses', by which he principally meant the clientele at popular assemblies, preferred set dances choreographed by British dancing masters. If the 'masses' did dance a Tango or Foxtrot, then it was typically in a re-named sequence version arranged by a home instructor.

In his presidential address to the BATD in 1914, J. D. McNaughton had observed that the 'commercial and professional classes' who patronised his members in contrast to the Boston Club of the Waldorf Hotel were not of the 'taste and temperament' to pursue 'a dance of such intricacy' as the Tango.[15] The matter was, in part, an economic one. Confusion over the many choreographed versions of the Tango, put out by separate teaching organizations, was leading to loss of public confidence in the profession. On the other hand, ready-made dances, new choreographies annually authorized by the teaching organizations, ensured a committed clientele who, following the same rhythm and pathways, could be packed in greater numbers into the hall. Taking issue with New York teacher Louis Chalif's observation that dancers no longer followed the dictates of teachers, McNaughton remonstrated that on the contrary 'the teacher must be the drillmaster'. No upper-middle-class dancer, however, would follow a drill set by a tradesperson. The opportunity to demonstrate initiative and quick thinking in sport was regarded as the birthright of the aristocratic and upper-middle-class male, who had been largely schooled on the playing fields of England rather than in the mindless physical education drill meted out to the working classes.

The upper-middle classes also relished their freedom to participate in a cosmopolitan culture. 'English Society', Richardson later observed,

> will not accept a ready-made dance, invented by a teacher. It will only act to novelties that have been thoroughly tested in New York or Paris'.[16]

The officer class (though now fewer in number in post-war London), those dancing enthusiasts of the Royalist Club, the Public Schools and Universities Club and their ilk, would not be dictated to by their social inferiors: they wanted a new dance in a 'fluid' state so that it may be 'developed or simplified', upon which they might imprint their own individuality, not conform as a *petit bourgeois*. Among Richardson's class of dancers, the call for standardization was not concerned with regulated dances, but with 'the teaching of definite and uniform base steps by all teachers, to which steps individual dancers may add as they please'.[17]

At the conclusion of hostilities in 1918, the first war ever to be conducted on a global scale had resulted in the rise of a new world order and a shift firmly away from the old royalist and patrician governance of Europe in which dancing had been so firmly embedded. War-time rhetoric had frequently focused on calls to defend civilization, but wartime experiences had equally confirmed that there could be no going back to Victorian convention.[18] A new order in the ballroom needed to be imposed on a population that sought escapism from the horrors of war in dancing and who continued to flock to the new cheaper and attractive *palais de danses* that had sprung up across towns and cities in Britain to cater for the rising number of lower-middle and working-class dancers and who were to dominate social dancing by the mid 1920s (Nott, 2002; McMains, 2006, pp. 80–4; Abra, 2009).

By the end of the war, the Boston and Tango had faded from the floor, replaced by the One-step, Hesitation Waltz, and Foxtrot. Differences between them might sometimes only be distinguished by the music, rather than by any discrete steps or style; even disciplinarian Scott (1920, p. 143) suggested that dancers might substitute *'bona fide* waltz steps' to the 4/4 of the Foxtrot. Many post-war dancers, however, eschewed identifiable dance steps by walking rhythmically to the music, responding bodily to the improvisatory nature of jazz music. A person of 'good taste' avowed Scott, however, would avoid dips, pumping the arms up and down, shaking the shoulders or swaying the hips. This appeal to good taste was to be echoed by Richardson that year when he called together the dance teaching profession to take the lead in restoring civilization to the ballroom, but in a modern guise.

Immersed in aristocratic codes of bodily conduct, the Society dancing master's *raison d'être* of course was the very act of corporeal refinement: dancing to jazz, the 'music of the jungle' was beyond the pale. This latest American musical import too, however, was later to be subject to processes of Europeanization. At the Grafton Galleries in 1920, it was reported that dance music for the coming season was to be 'smooth and tuneful' unlike the 'queer noises' of the American jazz band, the Versatile Four.[19] The 'nigger bands' whom Richardson believed to be unlikely to play a good Waltz tune were eventually to be replaced by predominantly white orchestras who, on mainly stringed instruments, specialized in 'symphonic syncopation' and later in strict tempo.[20] The initial task of the dancing profession, however, was to take control in restoring grace to the ballroom and to capitalize upon the nationwide enthusiasm for social dancing. In this it was enthusiastically supported by the popular press who characterized West End dancing as consisting of unexpected lifts and halts, rapid turning, couples suddenly veering across the path of others, and various versions of different dances to the same tune. 'The fact of the matter is ...' complained *The Daily Sketch*,

> modern dancing has no regulation steps: it is go-as-you-please dancing, an art into which each dancer is entitled to introduce any eccentric extravagance he fancies at the moment.[21]

Towards the modern English style

The initiative came from Maurice Mouvet, then performing in London, who wrote to Richardson suggesting that he called together the 'first-class dancing teachers of London' to discuss how ballroom dancing might be standardized among dancers of the more respectable establishments. Stressing dignity, as an ideal and existing attribute of the English, Maurice eschewed any presumption on his part to dictate to the 'Dancing World.' He had already led a similar venture in New York, but it was to be the English, with Richardson at the helm, who would steer ballroom dancing out of the chaotic seas of eclectic personal improvisation and contradictory and competitive teaching.[22]

Alert to the sensitivities of the profession, having long agitated for a centralizing national body, Richardson invited applications from any interested teacher to the tactfully named *informal* conference at the prestigious Grafton Galleries in May 1920. The event drew around two hundred teachers, the more well known, predominantly from London, but they also came from the provinces and colonies of South Africa and Ireland. Richardson ensured a strong media presence, sealing interest in the event with a performance and lecture-demonstration from Maurice and his partner Leonora Hughes (see Figure 17.1).[23]

Richardson's address at the conference drew artistic and politico-temporal comparisons, casting the move towards standardization as a revolt against the excesses of modernity and classicism. Led by fashionable dancers, he argued, the freedoms of the fashionable repertoire such as the Foxtrot and One-Step stood in opposition to the nineteenth-century style sequence dances of the old-fashioned dancing teachers. He went on to draw parallels with the Ballets Russes' professed modernizing agenda against the traditionalism of the ballet of the European opera houses.[24] His criticisms of contemporary social dancing drew on the long-established notion of the dance floor as a scaled-down mirror

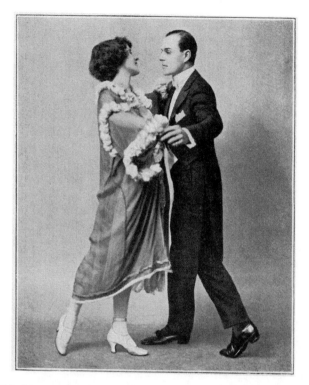

Figure 17.1 Maurice and Leonora Hughes, The Crossing Step in the Ballroom Fox-Trot, *The Dancing Times*, April 1920

of society. Tellingly, he saw political analogies in the recent war and the rise of communism:

> In the same way that in the great world of which the dancing world is but a microcosm, the free nations have revolted against the military autocracy of the Teutonic peoples. On the other hand, freedom from "sequence dances" must not mean that all law and order is to be jettisoned – that a species of dancing-Bolshevism is to be seen in our ballrooms.[25]

The way forward was not that of *petit bourgeois* dull and backward-looking conformity, but of upper-middle-class progressive, yet significantly moderate, modernity. Furthermore, Richardson was convinced that good taste would prevail: 'this feeling which exists among Englishmen and Englishwomen to do only that which is good form'.[26]

Quelling the anti-Americanism that arose on Maurice's departure from the conference, Richardson successfully chaired the meeting to a favourable vote: 'that the teachers present agree to do their very best to stamp out freak steps particularly dips and steps in which the feet are raised high off the ground and also sidesteps and pauses which impeded the progress of those who may be following.'[27] Scott, the mover of the motion, also succeeded in a rider that recommended side-steps to be taken at forty-five degrees to the line of dance in order to facilitate onward progression around the room. The conference then agreed to appoint a small committee to work on the more specific standardization of steps which was to report back to a general meeting in the autumn of 1920.

By the following May, three informal conferences had taken place in total, each organized and chaired by Richardson (1946). At the second, the basic steps of the One-Step, Foxtrot, and Tango had been agreed; at the third, there were additions and clarifications to the Foxtrot and Tango and agreement that the basic Waltz step which had tended towards a loss of identity should in future consist of 'step-step-feet together'. More fundamentally with respect to the modern technique was the suggestion that 'the knees must be kept together in passing and the feet parallel' (Richardson, 1946, p. 47). This means of progression around the dance floor, as if walking, was to lead to the modern English style's fundamental technique of placing the heel down first.

The informal conferences, followed by the detailed work undertaken by fashionable dancing teachers, were the first successful national attempts to standardize modern dancing in England, aided by *The Dancing Times*, a supportive press, and role models selected in competition and exhibition dancing. By the end of the decade, a distinctly modern English style of ballroom had been fashioned, led from 1924 by the ballroom branch of the ISDT. Leading teachers had favoured the ISDT, which Richardson had recommended others join, in order to become the undisputed majority ready to take on the detailed work of standardization. Essentially, the major elements of the style were already in place by 1920, indeed earlier in the graceful dancing of the Castles and of Oscar and Maurice Mouvet.

The torso was to move as an unbroken block: that meant no rotation of the pelvis, or moving it from side to side or sent back and forth; the shoulders were to be held straight and down, with no hunching and no movement back and forth, especially rapidly as indicated by the term 'shimmy'. The centre of gravity was to be held high, the weight transferred evenly and over the ball of the foot, the head held upright, never dropped, nor moved side to side, nor shaken. All movement quality was to be smooth, excluding sudden, jerky or angular movements. Above all, dancing was to be restrained, never demonstrative of excitement or displaying emotion. This was civilized dancing, redolent of the aristocratic aesthetic of bodily control and refinement, now fully in the hands of the upper-middle class and disseminated for those interested in genteel dancing further down the social scale. Rejected by London's West End, sequence dancing was soon to decline during the 1920s in a more democratic yet still very class-conscious society, keen to ape the repertoire of a fashionable world no longer led by the court, yet whose dancers in the modern *palais de danses* continued to buy into the code of gentility in the ballroom.

The embodiment of Englishness – in its guise of the civilized moderate Englishman and Englishwoman, able to recognize and practise principles of taste and good form – lay at the core of the transformation. It was an ideal shared by West End dancing teachers, in part if not always totally by Society and its upper-middle-class aspirants, and by many within the upwardly mobile lower-middle and upper-working classes who embraced such concepts fed to them though the press, Pathé news, the cinema, literature, and education. It was an ideal through which Richardson and the ISDT could achieve a social dance culture that embraced modernity within traditionally British aristocratic notions of civilization. As Richardson proudly proclaimed in the preface to his 1946 history of modern English ballroom dancing:

> England has undoubtedly taken the lead in the development of modern ballroom dancing. Other countries may have supplied the raw material and the dancers of New York, being nearer the source of that material, may have been the first to experiment with it, but it was the teachers of England who first analysed the crude steps, reduced order out of chaos and evolved the modern technique which has made the English style paramount over three-fifths of the globe.

That it could do so owed much to nineteenth-century foundations in a populous yet small nation that could still wield a worldwide imperial reach. In the process of standardization, a spatial hierarchy in which London, more specifically, the West End, was confirmed as the centralizing force over the provinces and the Commonwealth. This controlled dominance was in many respects a continuation of the existing centrifugal pull of the once imperial capital, accentuated by the commanding influence of socially well-connected members in national institutions such as *The Dancing Times* and the ISDT.

Through excellent communications in transport and media, and through its assured position of a refined bastion of cosmopolitan modernity, London gained hegemonic and often direct control over the provincial and the colonial. The London Style became synonymous with the English or British style and with missionary zeal, its teachers and dancers, often through branches of the Imperial Society of Teachers of Dancing, were to continue to visit the fading Empire.[28] By taking the lead in hosting world competitions, judged by leading West End teachers rather than by musical theatre stars, London became a magnet for the best in the profession. The style of quintessential English cool, the English gentleman and gentlewoman, became internationally desirable; it is significant to note that the American Fred Astaire modelled his dancing on Englishman Vernon Blyth, more famously known as Vernon Castle.

18
Looking Back, Moving On

> [W]here I am hoping to see the old style and the new
> style 'get together'.
>
> P. J. S. Richardson, *The Dancing Times*,
> June 1921, p. 703

In the post-First World War discourse on ballroom dancing technique, there is a marked emphasis on principles of simplicity, naturalness, and modernity, alongside and dovetailing with traditional values of refinement, civilization, and gentility. Moves away from complexity and artifice towards a more accessible and open style of moving were perceived at the time as symptomatic of the state of modernity. They also reflect a stylistic preference for a sparer clarity and elegance that resonates with other artistic developments, typically categorized under the umbrella of modernism.

The self-identified 'modern' stewards of fashionable dance culture increasingly professionalized dancing through the institutions and apparatus of competitions, occupational organizations, examinations, syllabuses, and a specialist press. In this process, some individuals felt a deep sense of loss, especially among the elite ranks of the high-class dancing teachers. Louis D'Egville (1917) was convinced that the root cause of the fall of civilized dancing lay in failure of public respect for the once powerful position of royal pedagogue and of the decline in attention to deportment. Turning his back on the dance floor, D'Egville focused his knowledge and creativity towards the theatre, and left the social arena of dancing in which he and his family had once held the highest position in the land. Unlike several generations before him, D'Egville's children did not follow in the family calling. After the First World War, he and, once arch rival, Mrs Wordsworth discovered that they had much in common.

As his conservative-minded son observed, the two were 'relics of the age of courtesy and dignity, an island in a turgid sea of jazz and Negroid wobblings' (D'Egville, 1937, p. 6).

Edward Scott, working into his late seventies, continued to harangue devotees of modern dancing, finding comfort and work from the dancing of the past and never reneging on his racist views that all evils of modern dancing stemmed from African culture. That social dancing, its practice, dissemination, and status in Britain had changed during these dancing masters' life times cannot be denied; yet, others with roots in Victorian dance culture, most notably Belle Harding, seized the call to modernize and built influential careers lasting well beyond the First World War. The demands of change, whether viewed as positive or degenerative, may have been uppermost in their minds; yet, there was often a conscious and creative search for continuities with the past in the name of modernity.

The emergence of the modern English ballroom style is typical of art historian Lynda Nead's (2000, p. 8) characterization of modernity as

> a set of processes and representations that were engaged in an urgent and inventive dialogue with their own historical conditions of existence.

To understand that development, it is beneficial for the dance historian to engage with larger trajectories of time and to view dancing, not only as interrelated genres that might appear across differing social contexts, but also as culturally embodied movement codes whose categorization needs to be addressed from the perspectives of contemporaneous voices.

For the majority of the twentieth century, mainstream dance historiography has favoured the radical over the conservative, the new over the old, novelty over tradition, and change over continuity. Perhaps this has been inevitable given the more professional formulation of dance historiography in the early years of that century, when the trajectories of modernism were integral to twentieth-century dance history's design and practice. In the wake of the cultural turn in dance historiography, Foucaldian-inspired analyses of dance history have further emphasized change, albeit more distinctly as rupture and discontinuity. Modernist and postmodernist approaches to dance history, however, which focus on tracing cultural changes rather than continuities, may obscure potential for exploring deeper historical processes at work. Limited consideration of socio-cultural continuities in dance threatens appreciation of social and cultural agency in the maintenance, creativity, and dissemination of dance practices.

This initial investigation of Society dancing in England across the late-nineteenth and early-twentieth centuries has dipped into numerous channels for deeper and more extensive navigation. Seeking to understand more of the social production of dancing and of its agents across this time frame has necessarily brought into view well-established issues in dance scholarship, but which hopefully in future may be approached from perspectives other than those derived from the dominant focus upon European concert dance. These issues tantalizingly form a complex of clusters which, for the purposes of analysis, often prove difficult to untangle. These include, in particular, the decline of dancing as an integral aspect of socio-political activities within Eurocentric contexts; the growing separation of amateur and professional spheres; the status of the dancing man, sexuality and the performative construction of national character; the play of intergenerational leadership in the acceptance and disavowal of dance practices; and the institutionalization and feminization of dance across a number of dance genres. More detailed study of relations between modernity and modernism within the realm of the social and the popular also promises greater insight into later conceptualizations, values, and practices of dancing in Britain.

Notions of modernity and modernism are, of course, by no means singular; nor, indeed, do such categorizations relate to strict chronological order (Osborne, 1992). From the mid to late-nineteenth century, many people living in Britain were conscious that they were living in modern times, an appraisal which, in the fast-moving world of easier communications and increasing centralization, strengthened, and quickened towards the First World War. During this period, experiences of modernity, qualitative and relational, differed geographically, socially, and individually (Daunton and Rieger, 2001), but in urban and cosmopolitan contexts, comparisons with the past, whether adverse or positive, were more acute and voluble.

As Society gradually yielded its influential character, laments on the passing of a more ordered, peer-inclusive and choreographically diverse experience on the Society dance floor, acted as a refrain in the discourse on fashionable social dancing. Not surprisingly they were loudest among those who stood to lose power in their cultural sphere, notably high-class dancing teachers and Society hostesses. At their extreme, such protestations against change interpreted the new habits of modern times as evidence of degeneration, the sure symptoms of the decline of civilization. For these critics looking back to a supposedly more civilized age, the quotidian rate of change appeared an accelerating and uncontrollable force. In the eyes of conservative contemporaries, the sense of speed had permeated the *fin de siècle* dance floor, manifest in the quickening tempo of the Waltz and in the romping style of the Lancers. The slower pace of the past felt increasingly out of reach for Society dancing. Even the conservative and hopeful ISDT dancing teachers doubted the efficacy of the historical dance revival. Modern life was now 'too quick in these motoring days to reacquire the old grace and stateliness'.[1]

Nonetheless, modernity as a positive force in social dancing gained precedence, though the precise meaning and usage of the term were variable. In the late nineteenth century, Victorian dancing masters, such as Crompton and Scott, had described their own teaching methods, style, and compositions as modern. Ever anxious to be abreast of changing fashion and to court respect for the profession, they adopted the descriptor to signal their work as scientific, systematic, and up-to-date. In the early 1910s, the concept of 'modern dancing' differentiated the style and repertoire of post-ragtime dances from the staid proprieties of the Victorian past and from the perceived indelicacies of an African-American and lower-class present. By the 1920s, the notion of modern social dancing embraced similar affiliations, with emphasis upon 'naturalness', 'gentility' and 'Englishness'. In light of this complex of meanings, future studies might usefully integrate analysis of the discourse of theatrical dancing and of other forms of culturally codified movement to achieve greater critical understanding of the emergence of distinctive twentieth-century dance genres, as well as a more rounded appreciation of the period.

From the early 1910s, transformation from dominance of the centuries-old aristocratic European aesthetic on the fashionable dance floor to one inflected with African-American and European lower-class bodily codes wrought major and, in many respects, irreversible changes on the social dance culture of fashionable Britain. That transition, however, was not an abrupt revolution, nor was its effect immediate across the population. Lynda Nead (2000, p. 8) has fruitfully drawn upon Michel Serres's evocative metaphor of the crumpled handkerchief in which the experience of modernity may be considered as 'pleated or crumpled time, drawing together past, present and future into constant and unexpected relations'. That sense of multitemporalities, of past, present, and future is evident from the records of dancing in the years subsequent to Nead's interdisciplinary analysis of London in the mid-nineteenth century. Characteristic of the experience of modernity in the dance culture of the late Victorian and Edwardian years is the revival of historical and so-called folk dances. Although suffused by dissatisfaction with contemporary aspects of modern life, the trawl of the past in these seemingly backward-looking movements for cultural models to revivify the present and to build foundations for the future, was not entirely the nostalgic prerogative of an older generation. The revivals did not, as noted above, succeed in convincing the whole population to look back, whether in old books or in the supposedly static countryside, in order to move forwards on the social dance floor, but they each did attract a committed amateur following.[2] Less easily discernible, but more closely attached to ball room dancing, were the opportunities for a diversity of practices within a populous, heterogeneous, and mobile society. Deviations from the ideal kinetic paradigm were in evidence, even among the fashionable, well before the advent of ragtime in London. In the Kensington Crawl of the 1880s, the early Boston, the Two-Step, and One-Step,[3] indeed, in the ways in which people often muddled their way in a pedestrian manner around the dance floor, might be viewed moments of individualism and of small group activity that suggest new ways of moving, but which ebbed back before the later greater tide of American imports. Rather than the analogy of a crumpled handkerchief, the modernity of London's dance culture might be viewed as a waterscape, open to the ever-moving sea, bringing and taking new elements, harbouring quiet backwaters, deep channels, cross-currents, surging waves and moments of extreme turbulence.[4]

Metaphors may help in approaching complex phenomena, but it is important not to lose the specificity of agency and space in seeking to theorise dance practices from socio-cultural perspectives. The dangers of reductionism and determinism are ever present, threatening to oust recognition of the visceral enjoyment of dancing from our understanding. At this distance, when the voices are long stilled, the means to access testimonies of those bodily sensations are inevitably limited. Even so, notes of caution may be sounded from the archive in the effort to avoid further traps of presentist projection and all-inclusive theory.

In identifying and aligning aspects of age, gender, class, and race with distinctive dance practices, there have emerged individuals in the course of this investigation who, despite their background and seeming set of circumstances, fly in the face of the emerging norm: at the end of the nineteenth century, for example, the enthusiasm of certain aristocratic and upper-class men for dancing belies the growing expectation that men of social station do not dance. For every young debutante that yearned to be swept into the Waltz, there were also those who hated the Season's dances, preferring instead (though occasionally as well as) the experience of riding to hounds, playing lawn tennis, or studying classics. Not all young people rushed to dance ragtime and Tango, but instead embraced historical and folk dances with a passion that carried them throughout their lives. Just as the experience of modernity cannot be condensed to a single chronological category, neither can individual cultural expression be explained solely by social and cultural factors.

What has clearly emerged in this study, however, as an identifiable social trend from the late nineteenth century, is the flourishing of dance as a democratized leisure activity, an activity of personal choice rather than social duty. The growing array of different genres from past and present and from other continents that increasingly appeared on offer to a greater number of participants, presented more diverse options for self-expression and for potential affiliation with social groups often removed from an individual's position at birth. It is a feature that becomes especially prominent in the latter part of the twentieth century when individuals had scope to identify with dance and music practices that today circulate globally. This mobility was already evident in the late nineteenth and early twentieth centuries as communications opened up new possibilities to a growing urban and more affluent population. Similarly, the shift away from artifice towards a more 'natural' manner of dancing as social interaction and towards individual expression, especially of the young, runs as a leitmotif into mainstream popular dance activities of twentieth-century Britain.

In looking back and moving on, it is hoped that this investigation of dancing among Britain's Society during the late nineteenth and early twentieth centuries may sound a rallying call; first, to re-assert the value of and to renew, with fresh eyes, detailed and extensive activity in the archives; second, to address continuity as well as change within the practice of dance historiography, and, finally, above all, to demonstrate the historian's creed that without knowledge of our pasts we can neither know our presents, nor prepare for our futures.

Appendix: Key Personnel in Society Dancing in England 1870–1920

This appendix is merely indicative of some of the principal personalities, referred to in this book, who played a key role in transmitting and shaping Society dancing. There is, as yet, no database of individuals working in dance during this period in Britain and the listing below serves merely to provide a quick reference for readers. Details on the lives of Society dancing teachers remain comparatively sparse. Further information on the personnel below may be sought in the notes, bibliography, and index and, for the more luminous examples, in the *ODNB*.

Royalty and Society

Edward VII, born Albert Edward (1841–1901), the Prince of Wales officiated for Queen Victoria at state balls, following the death of his father, the Prince Consort Albert in 1861. Once an avid dancer himself, he later restricted his dancing primarily to the opening ceremonial Quadrille of the evening.

Queen Alexandra (1844–1925) Princess Alexandra of Denmark, formerly known as the Princess of Wales, wife of Edward VII, Prince of Wales, was noted for her love of dancing, particularly the Waltz. She was an influential leader of fashion and deportment.

Queen Mary (1867–1953) née the Princess of Teck and known to her family as May, Mary was noted, as the wife of George V, for her regal deportment, instilled no doubt by childhood lessons with Taglioni and D'Egville.

Ancaster, Lady, Countess of Ancaster (1846–1921) née Evelyn Elizabeth Gordon, daughter of the Marquess of Huntly, Lady Ancaster married into the Heathcote-Drummond-Willoughby family and was a noted Society leader who was known as the Countess of Ancaster from 1892 to 1910. She contributed to Lilly Grove's *Dancing* (1895), *The Morning Post*, and *The Dancing Times* and was a recognized authority on standards of Society dancing.

Asquith, Cynthia (1887–1960) née Lady Cynthia Charteris, daughter of the Earl of Wemyss, she was a novelist and diarist whose memoirs (*Haply I May Remember*, 1950 and *Remember and Be Glad*, 1952) include observations on 'coming out' and lessons with Louis D'Egville and Mrs Wordsworth.

Asquith, Margot (1864–1945) née Margaret Tennant, daughter of an industrialist and politician, she became a member of the intellectual set known as 'The Souls' and married the future Prime Minister Herbert Asquith. Her autobiography includes memories of her own dancing experiences.

Churchill, Lady Randolph (1854–1921), daughter of an American businessman, Jennie Jerome married into English aristocracy and is best known today as the mother of Winston Churchill. As Mrs Cornwallis-West (her second marriage following the death of Lord Randolph), she was very active in instigating and promoting the Shakespeare fancy dress ball (1911) and performed at the piano for Nellie Chaplin's historical music and dance concerts.

Esher, Viscount (1852–1930) Reginald Baliol Brett, historian and Liberal politician, was educated at Eton and Trinity College, Cambridge. A keen dancer at Society balls, his memoirs were published as *Cloud-Capp'd Towers*.

Greville, Lady Violet (1842–1932) née Beatrice Violet Graham, daughter of the Duke of Montrose, Lady Greville wrote *The Gentlewoman in Society* (1892) and co-authored the 'Place aux Dames' column for the *Daily Graphic*. As well as short essays on dance, she composed novels and produced various articles and an edited book on ladies' sport.

Armytage, Hon. Mrs (1832–1903) née Fenella Fitzhardinge Berkeley, a baron's daughter. Mrs Armytage was the author of *Old Court Customs and Modern Court Rule* (1883) and mother of Society master of ceremonies, Percy Armytage.

Armytage, Percy (1853–1934). Educated at Wellington College and King's College School, Percy Armytage became the first professional Society master of ceremonies and later gentleman usher to Edward VII and George V. A composer of waltzes, he offers first-hand information on royal and Society balls in his memoirs, *By the Clock of St James's* (1927).

Marlborough, Duchess of (1877–1964). Daughter of the rich American Vanderbilt family, Consuelo Vanderbilt became Duchess of Marlborough on her marriage to Charles Spencer-Churchill. Schooled in dancing and deportment by New York Society dancing master Allen Dodworth, she offers interesting observations on English court ceremony and dancing in her memoirs *The Glitter and the Gold* (Balsan, 1953).

Richardson, Constance Stewart, Lady (1883–1932). Daughter of the Earl of Cromartie and niece of the Duke of Sutherland, Constance was a champion swimmer, big-game hunter, and classical (i.e. Greek-inspired) dancer who took to the professional stage. Reviews of her performances were mixed and Philip Richardson noted improvement after lessons in classical ballet. She wrote *Dancing, Beauty and Games* (1913).

Rolfe, Margaret A. B. (1873–1962). Child pupil of Marie Taglioni, Margaret Rolfe's reminiscences and drawings of this family friend and of her lessons from 1876 to 1880 in London are contained in *The Book of Marie Taglioni*, held in the Theatre and Performance Collection at the Victoria and Albert Museum.

Society teachers of dancing

Crompton, Robert (c. 1844–1926). Initiator and editor of the first specialist dance periodical, *Dancing* (1891–1893) in England, Crompton was a prominent activist for the profession. He was based in London from the 1880s, as a choreographer and trainer of dancers for stage and salon, enjoying international recognition. He was one of the prime movers and first President of the Imperial Society of Dance Teachers (ISDT, later the Imperial Society of Teachers of Dancing).

D'Albert, Charles (18??–1923). Teacher of dancing from the mid 1870s and of the Delsarte method of physical culture from the 1890s, D'Albert was the first

Vice President and Honorary Secretary of the ISDT. Editor of *The Dance Journal* and European correspondent to *The Two Step*, he was noted for his knowledge of dance history. In 1913, he published the *Technical Encyclopaedia of the Theory and Practice of the Art of Dancing* (revised 1921) and contributed to *The Dancing Times*.

D'Egville, Louis (1819–1892). A member of the famous D'Egville dynasty of dancers and teachers, Louis was a founder member of 'The Wandering Minstrels' amateur orchestra and noted violinist who kept company with eminent musicians of the day. He jealously guarded the lineage as royal dancing master which reputedly stretched back to the court at Versailles.

D'Egville, Louis (1857–1927). Son of Louis and nephew of Mme Michau, with both of whom he worked, Louis D'Egville, the younger, tutored royalty and aristocracy at his home in Conduit Street, central London. A composer and violinist as well as teacher of dancing, deportment, and court presentation, he later taught at the Academy of Dramatic Art.

Garratt, Elizabeth. Born in 1859, she was a former pupil of Taglioni and a niece of Mme Stainton Taylor. Elizabeth came to prominence as a teacher of Society children in the 1890s. The *Pall Mall Gazette* ran a feature on her popular At Homes in Kensington where she featured exhibitions of skirt, historical, and other fancy dancing.

Harding, Isabella (c.1865–1945). Belle Harding was a prominent teacher of new Society dances in the first half of the twentieth century. Responsible for introducing tango tea dances into London hotels, she was quick to promote new trends and offered an extensive teaching and pedagogic training system throughout Britain and the northern French coastal resorts.

Henderson, Nicholas, Mr (c.1818–1891) and Mrs (née Frances Bonton, c.1821–1878), together with their daughter Elizabeth (born 1841) were based in Newman Street, Marylebone, and regularly advertised in *The Times*. Mrs Henderson brought out several editions of her ballroom guide.

Humphrey, Edward (1839–1918). Edward established the London Academy of Dancing in Cavendish Square, London, in 1863, which specialized in Society and fancy dancing. He was the author of several editions of *The London Ball Room Guide* and founding editor of the first series of *The Dancing Times* 1894–1902.

Humphrey, Walter E. (1866–1922). Walter was the Chief Instructor at his father's London Academy of Dancing and creator of numerous Society dances. He also produced an edition of *The London Ball Room Guide* (1900) and contributed various articles on fashionable dances to the second series of *The Dancing Times*.

Johnson, Henry R. Born c. 1864, Johnson was a teacher of dancing, together with his wife, Frances, at Tavistock Place and Edgware Road, London. A popular Master of Ceremonies, especially at Covent Garden, the Portman Rooms and Holborn Town Hall during the 1890s, he was a founding member and a later President of the BATD.

Lamb, William. Proprietor of the South London School of Dancing and an early president of the BATD, Lamb was the author of *Everybody's Guide to Ball-Room Dancing* [1896] and *How and What to Dance* (1904).

Lennard, Janet, Miss. Instrumental in promoting the Boston in the West End through the Keen Dancers Society in the early 1900s, Janet Lennard contributed articles on ballroom dancing to *The Dancing Times* in the early years of its second series.

Michau, Caroline D'Egville, Mme (c. 1821–1892). Niece of the 'celebrated Mme Michau' (née Sophia D'Egville, brother of James, choreographer and ballet master at the King's Theatre earlier in the century), Caroline married her first cousin, dancing master James Paul Michau (c. 1822–1883). A teacher in Brighton and London Society circles, she composed both music and dances and published a treatise on deportment and dancing in 1861.

Piaggio, Francis (1838–1914). A founding member of the BATD, Piaggio was noted for his dances at Margate and for the well-attended St Patrick, St Andrew, and St George's night balls which he ran at the Portman Rooms. Many a young man began his dancing experience in the shilling hops at 'Piggies'.

Scott, Edward (1852–1937). Based for much of his long career in Brighton and Hove on the south coast, Scott was a recognized authority on ball room dancing technique and on dance history. He was the author of numerous books, articles and letters on dance but remained fiercely opposed to styles prevalent among the working class and those dances introduced from African-American culture.

Stainton Taylor, Mme (1831–1900). Born Elizabeth Stainton, she regularly advertised her South Kensington School of Dancing in *The Times* and other Society press, offering lessons in callisthenics, deportment, ballroom dancing, court presentation, and skirt dancing.

Taglioni, Marie (1804–1884). The most famous ballerina of her generation, Taglioni in later life taught deportment, court presentation, and dancing mostly to the upper echelons of British society in London during the 1870s.

Vacani, Marguerite, Mme. Listed in British telephone books from 1908 as a teacher of dancing based in the West End, Marguerite Vacani (born 1885) was the daughter of an immigrant Italian family dealing in fine art and furniture. She assiduously courted an aristocratic clientele, eventually becoming tutor to the royal family. The Vacani School of Dancing, later continued by her niece Betty Vacani, was responsible for many a debutante's presentation at court.

Wordsworth, Mrs (1843–1932). Born Isabella Annie Wordsworth to a Brighton family of dancing teachers, Mrs Wordsworth became the most celebrated Society teacher of dancing and deportment in the 1890s and early 1900s. Her system of teaching and cultural cachet attracted numerous young women of social standing into the dancing profession, some of whom, to her great distaste, went on to perform on the stage.

Performers and theatre personnel

Bradley, Josephine (1893–1985). A champion ballroom dancer in the 1920s, Josephine Bradley played an influential role in the early and subsequent years of the ISTD ballroom branch and helped to establish the English style.

Castle, Irene (née Foote, 1893–1969) and Vernon (né Vernon Blyth 1887–1918) were an English husband and American wife team of exhibition ballroom dancers and teachers who rose to international fame following performances in Paris and New York. Elegant and graceful, they promoted tasteful dancing of the new repertoire (publishing *Modern Dancing* in 1914) and earned extraordinarily high salaries and international celebrity status before Vernon's fatal flying accident in 1918. Fred Astaire and Ginger Rogers later played the couple in a tribute film.

De Rhynal, Camille. Dancer, choreographer, and teacher, De Rhynal organized Tango competitions in Nice and Paris and played an important role in the establishment of world dance championships.

Grossmith, George (1847–1912). Actor, singer, entertainer, writer. Educated at the North London Collegiate School, George Grossmith is best known today for his performance of numerous Gilbert and Sullivan roles and for his literary creation of Pooter in *The Diary of a Nobody*. A multi-talented entertainer, he composed and performed satirical songs, many of which provide insight into English manners and dancing. An excellent dancer himself, his observations on Society fashion and on dancing were often sought by the press.

Grossmith, George, Junior (1874–1935). Following his father into the theatre, George Grossmith Junior, became an actor, singer, dancer, playwright, director, theatre producer, and manager. He was known especially in musical comedies for his comic characterization of upper-class brainless young men. Enjoying a reputation as a fashionable man about town, Grossmith's performances of the Argentine Tango with Phyllis Dare in *The Sunshine Girl* (1912) helped to popularize the dance. His actor brother Lawrence married the sister of Vernon Castle.

Mouvet, Maurice (1888–1927). Born in New York to Belgian parents, Maurice's fame as an international exhibition ballroom dancer rivalled that of the Castles, whom he regarded as having usurped his premier position. Dancing first with his wife Florence Walton, later with his second wife Leonora Hughes, his performances of the Apache, Tango, and his solo Skating Waltz in particular were widely imitated. He was instrumental, together with Philip Richardson, in galvanizing the English ballroom dancing profession after the war.

Mouvet, Oscar. The elder brother of Maurice, Oscar was one of the very first exhibition ballroom dancers to appear in London in 1911, initially with his partner Regine and then with Suzette. Greatly admired by Philip Richardson for his graceful yet manly dancing, Oscar left the stage after the war to become a Parisian restaurant owner.

Silvester, Victor (1900–1978). Initially trained by Belle Harding, clergyman's son Victor Silvester went on to become one of the most famous names in English ballroom dancing. An influential member of the early ISTD ballroom branch, he wrote a number of books on ballroom dancing technique and, as bandleader, his brand of strict tempo music, regularly transmitted on BBC radio, made his a household name.

Vaughan, Kate (?1852–1903) née Catherine Candelon, daughter of a musician, Kate was trained in ballet by Mme Conquest and later by John D'Auban. Famed for her refined and graceful skirt dancing, she was a favourite at the Gaiety Theatre and married (and divorced) the Hon. Frederick Wellesley. Ill health and ambition drove her later turn towards an acting career, for which she received some favourable reviews. Her ladylike dancing and deportment were rarely equalled by her successors in skirt dancing during the 1890s.

Writers on Dance

Grove, Lilly (c. 1855–1941) Born in France, Lilly Grove turned to writing to support herself and children in England on the death of her husband: the Badminton Library volume *Dancing* was published in 1895. She married the anthropologist Sir James Frazer in 1896.

Richardson, Philip John Sampey (1875–1963). Born into a Midlands brewing family, Richardson became a clerk and journalist in London, where in 1910 he established the title of *The Dancing Times* as the foremost professional dance journal. He was the propelling influential force behind much of Britain's dance infrastructure of the twentieth century: the ballroom branch of the ISTD, the Camargo Society, the Royal Academy of Dance, the Sunshine Competitions, the Official Board of Ballroom Dancing, and later the International Council of Ballroom Dancing. He authored *A History of English Ballroom Dancing* (1946) and *The Social Dances of the Nineteenth Century in England* (1960).

Notes

1 Fashionable Bodies and Society Dancing

1. On social mobility and the mutual influence of cultural habits in nineteenth-century England with respect to the middle and upper classes, see Thompson (1988); Bush (1984); Young (2003); James (2006).
2. See, for example, Hobsbawm (1987); Harris (1994); Pugh (1999); Searle (2004). On general dance history of the period, scholarship in which tends towards a North American bias, see Ruyter (1979); Erenberg (1981); Tomko (1999).
3. On historians' interpretations of the impact of the First World War see Constantine, Kirby, and Rose (1995).
4. For discussion on the nature of cultural history see Rubin (2002); Burke (2004); Mandler (2004a, 2004b); Hesse (2004); Jones (2004); Watts (2004); Green (2007).
5. On the development of London in the nineteenth century see Thorold (2001) and White (2007).
6. The seminal text on the London Season is Davidoff (1973). See also Evans and Evans (1976); Horn (1992).
7. See Beckett (1986); Cannadine (1996). These issues form recurrent motifs in post-First World War aristocratic autobiographies.
8. Anon. ([1874]), p. 3. Copy in Jerome Robbins Dance Division, New York Public Library.
9. My reading of social distinction and cultural capital among the English aristocracy and bourgeoisie draws much upon Elias (1978) and Bourdieu (1984).
10. For examples of social and cultural analysis using such sources see Morgan (1994) and St George (1993). For an invaluable online source of American and European dancing manuals, together with insightful commentary, see Aldrich (2005) http://memory.loc.gov/ammem/dihtml/dihome.html.
11. Philip J. S. Richardson, editor of the second series of *The Dancing Times*, provides a contemporary characterization of the relation of class, venue, time of year, and social context which is based on his own contribution to the first issue of the revamped journal in October 1910.
12. For the development of British leisure see Walton and Walvin (1983); Walton (1983); Lowerson (1993); Bailey (2003).
13. For discussion of these dance forms and their treatment in fictional literature of the period, see Engelhardt (2009); Wilson (2009); Thompson (1998). For related activities in Paris see Cordova (1999).

2 Fashioning Dance Histories

1. For overviews of popular, social and folk dancing see the respective entries in the *International Encyclopedia of Dance* (1998).

2. On the growing division between the theatrical and the social in Western European dance, see, for example, Cohen (2000) and McGowan (2008).
3. The division in dance historiography becomes crystallized during this period into the 1920s. Compare, for example, the organization and treatment of social and theatrical dancing in Grove (1895), Vuillier (1898), Scott (1899), St. Johnston (1906) and Urlin [1914] with Flitch (1912) and Kinney and Kinney (1914). The early twentieth century is witness to an increase in books on specific genres of dance. See, for example, Sharp (1907–13), Neal (1910), Coles [1909] and (1910), Chaplin (1911), Crozier [1913], Perugini (1915) and Johnson (1915).
4. For academia's focus upon European concert music see Stock (1998).
5. Key examples are Quirey (1976) and Buckman (1978).
6. See Kealiinohomoku (1969–70) reprinted several times, more recently in Dils and Albright (2001). For considerations of the 'cultural turn' in dance historiography, see Koritz (1996), Bryson (1997) and Carter (2004a and 2004b). The impact of the 'cultural turn' extends, of course, beyond the historiographical study of dance: see Morris (2009) and Buckland (2006).
7. Seminal texts are Foster (1995) and (1996). See also Thomas (2003). Historiographical approaches to dance as embodied cultural practice are now extensive in dance studies. For a more radical understanding of this approach, see Albright (2003–4).
8. On the critical need for interrogation of universalist understandings of the human body, see Farnell (1994) and, as example, Grau (2005).
9. For a critique of such approaches, see Brooks (2002). A more sympathetic overview is given in Carter (2004a).
10. The standard text on the methodology of dance history is Adshead-Lansdale and Layson (1994).
11. On the growth of the press in the late nineteenth century, see Vann and VanArsdel (1994), Brown (1985), and Brake (2001); on literacy, see Altick (1957).
12. On the development of a specialist press for women, see Ledbetter (2009).
13. *The Morning Post*, 16 July 1897. References to her letter can be found not only in the British media, but also in that of the United States: see *The Morning Post*, 27 July 1897 and *The Two Step*, 4, 38 (1897), 200, 213.
14. References to this journal follow those of the facsimile copy (Toronto: Press of Terpsichore, 1984). On Crompton's activities see Buckland (2007). I am most grateful to the former editor of *The Dancing Times*, Mary Clarke, and to her staff for access to the first series of the journal. Reference to *The Ball Room* is made in *The Dancing Times*, September 1901.
15. A key source was John Weaver's *An Essay Towards An History of Dancing* (1712). See Richard Ralph's scholarly edition (1985) of Weaver's works and his discussion of Weaver's influence.
16. On the production and consumption of etiquette books, see Young (2003). Lady Violet Greville (1892) also wrote the 'Place aux dames' column for the *Daily Graphic* and, as well as short essays on dance, produced various articles and an edited book on ladies' sport. See Armytage (1883) and for the activities of her son Percy, see Armytage (1927).
17. For more detail on the activities of dancing teachers see Chapters 7 and 8.
18. On the domestic use of music in the period and the wider socio-economic production and consumption of music see Ehrlich (1985) and Temperley (1989).

19. See Chapters 7 and 8 for further detail.
20. *Punch* artist Lewis Baumer, for example, was a member of a programme committee for dances in London in the early 1900s. On the principal *Punch* cartoonists who illustrated dance scenes, see Thorpe (1935), Houfe (2002), Kelly (1996), Engen (1991) and for Baumer, see entry in Bryant (2000).
21. Philip John Sampey Richardson (1875–1963), grandson of a prosperous Midlands brewer became a London-based clerk then writer and journalist. See entry in *Oxford Dictionary of National Biography* (hereafter *ODNB*) and Genné (1982). An in-depth examination of his contribution to British and international dance culture is long overdue.
22. For example, *The Dancing World* (copies in the British Library from October 1920), the monthly journal *The Dancer* edited by Espinosa (though his self-confident voice could not be called muted) and *The Ball Room*, a monthly periodical which also produced an annual publication *Dancing* (copies of the last two from the 1920s in my personal possession).

3 The Seasonal Round

1. There is extensive advice on giving dances but see, for example, Boyle (1873); *Lady's Pictorial* 2 July 1887, 9 July 1887, 1 October 1887; Campbell (1893); *Saturday Review* 2 April 1887; Armstrong [1900].
2. On the plutocracy and the Prince of Wales's set, see Cowles (1956).
3. See Chancellor (1908) and Pearce (2001). For illustrations of ball rooms see Devonshire House and Norfolk House (Chancellor, 1908, facing p. 231 and facing p. 313), Stafford House and Wimbourne House (Pearce, 2001, pp. 199, 209); staircases at Dorchester House (Chancellor, 1908, facing p. 249) Londonderry House and Stafford House (Pearce, 2001, pp. 159, 198). The last ball room to be added to a London mansion was Derby House in 1908 (Pearce, 2001). On the imitative building of the *nouveaux riches*, see Crook (1999).
4. These rules were, of course, breached from time to time. See Lovelace (1932, pp. 26–7) on restrictions placed on young Society women; see also Chapter 11.
5. *Dancing* April 1892, p. 131. See also Powell (1978).
6. 8 February. On his associations with Society, see Grossmith (1888).
7. On American heiresses, see Kehoe (2004), Balsan (1953), Armytage (1927) and Jennings (2007). Privileged American society shared similar rules of etiquette in the ball room with English Society; see Aldrich (1991, 2009).

4 Public Spaces

1. On procedures for public balls attended by Society, see, for example, A Member of the Aristocracy (1879).
2. For coverage of the Royal Caledonian Ball see, for example, *The Times* 30 June 1874, 20 June 1882, 13 May 1892.
3. On the growth of accommodation and hospitality to meet the rising number of affluent visitors to London, see Clayton (2005); Jackson and Nathan (2004); White (2007). See also contemporary listings in Pascoe (1897) and in the Baedeker guides to London.

4. The problem was familiar earlier in the century; see the fictional example in Marryat (1841).
5. *The Daily Telegraph*, 11 August 1899.
6. See, for example, *Dancing*, September 1891, p. 48 and March 1892, p. 118. For indication of the size of the Portman Rooms see illustration in *The Dancing Times* November 1912, p. 85.
7. See listings in the first series of *The Dancing Times* as well as advertisements for Society charity balls in *The Times*.
8. For satirical references to tradespeople at fashionable dances see 'Mixed Company' *Punch*, 23 September 1876 and 'At a Subscription Dance' *Punch*, 17 May 1899.
9. *The Dancing Times*, December 1899, p. 8.
10. *Dancing* published a series of articles, 'Metropolitan Dancing Halls and Assemblies' which nicely typifies the social gradation of middle-class public dances in London in the early 1890s. The Kensington Cinderellas held their 32nd season in 1912 (*The Dancing Times*, December, p. 177).
11. 'How to Run a Subscription Dance', October, pp. 5–7; *The Dancing Times*, November 1911, p. 38; *The Dancing Times*, October 1910, p. 20.
12. For the highly influential Harris, see *The Oxford Dictionary of National Biography* (ODNB); coverage and advertisements in *The Times*. See also Machray (1902).
13. *The Times*, 13 December 1895; *The Times*, 29 December 1897.
14. See, for example, coverage on the coronation season's balls in *The Dancing Times*, February, March, April, May and June 1911. For the Savoy's new ballroom, see cover illustration of this book and *The Dancing Times*, January 1911, pp. 82–4. For the Albert Hall, see *The Dancing Times*, December 1913, pp. 153–61.
15. See Chapter 10; also, for example, the appearance of theatrical people in costume at the fancy dress ball patronized by the Prince and Princess of Teck at the Savoy Hotel, *The Dancing Times*, April 1911, p. 196.

5   Late Victorian Repertoire

1. For a detailed study of the history and performance practices of the Quadrille, see Rogers (2003).
2. See, for example, The Caledonians in LeBlanc [1883], Crompton [1891], Lamb [1896], and Scott (1911).
3. Crompton [1891], Richardson (1960), LeBlanc [1883]; quotation from *Capel Court Chronicle* cited in LeBlanc [1883, pp. 50–1].
4. *Dancing*, June 1891, p. 1; Crompton [1891].
5. On the Waltz pre-1900, see Richardson (1960), Katz (1973), Knowles (2009) and especially for its earlier variations, of which there were many in the early 1800s, see Aldrich (1990) and Wilson (2009).
6. Descriptions of how the two steps were performed in the *Valse à Trois Temps* vary across the century, geographically and socially. Dutch dancing master Henri Dacunha (1872) working in London in the late 1860s notes that the dance was also known as the 'Hop Waltz' (the *deux pas* here appear to relate to a step on the first beat of the bar followed by a hop landing on the third

of the bar) and that a Galop step was often used in the *Valse à Deux Temps*. Other descriptions refer to the first step taking two beats. See also Aldrich (1990) for fuller discussion of other examples.

7. *The Times*, 5 July 1870.
8. See, for example, articles in *The Times*, 12 July 1877, 22 March 1878, 18 May 1882, 3 June 1886, 11 July 1891, 16 July 1895, 19 May 1899.
9. For contemporary descriptions of these dances see, for example, Humphrey [1874], Crompton [1891] and Lamb [1896]; for a chronological survey of *The Triumph* see Walker (2001).
10. As contemporary perception, see *The Dancing Times*, November 1902, p. 4.
11. See, for example, descriptions in LeBlanc [1883] and Scott (1911).
12. See, for example, descriptions in Scott (1911).
13. Comparatively few discrete notations of the Two-Step in late Victorian and Edwardian English dance manuals may be found, no doubt because most people merely adapted the turning of the Waltz to the music's 6/8 rhythm.
14. See, for example, the German state ball programme reproduced in *The Dance Journal*, March 1909, p. 2.

6 Anarchy in the Ball Room

1. *The Dancing Times*, March 1895, p. 8, December 1894, p. 7.
2. *The Dancing Times*, February 1895, p. 8.
3. *The Dancing Times*, December 1894, p. 7. Cf. correspondence in *The Morning Post* from Coppélia, 23 December 1898, Edward Lawson, 4 January 1899, Cyril A. Norris, 10 January 1899, Edward Scott, 6 February 1899.
4. A Glyder, *The Dancing Times*, March 1895, p. 8.
5. Ibid.
6. *The Dancing Times*, January 1911, p. 90.
7. *London and Brighton*, 16 March 1882.
8. *Pall Mall Gazette*, 7 February 1889.
9. *The Dancing Times*, September 1894, p. 3.
10. *Pall Mall Gazette*, 7 February 1889.
11. 'A Terrible Alternative', *Punch*, 10 January 1885.
12. *Judy*, 25 February 1880.
13. See cartoon in *Funny Folks*, 21 March 1885, following a report in *The Graphic* on the contemporary number of Waltz styles.
14. Consuelo Vanderbilt (Duchess of Marlborough) was puzzled by this rule since she and her American peers were regularly taught such a manoeuvre; see Balsan (1953). There may have been other less ostensible reasons: aesthetically and politically, a sovereign could look out on a roomful of subjects all turning the same way in harmony, or there may have lurked the old idea that to turn widdershins, i. e. anti-clockwise, portends evil.
15. 7 February.
16. *Pall Mall Gazette*, 7 February 1889.
17. Quoted in *The Dancing Times*, November 1902, pp. 2–3.
18. 23 January 1899.
19. Ibid.
20. *The Dancing Times*, November 1902, p. 3.

21. *The Morning Post*, 6 February 1899.
22. 25 September.
23. For details on the Messels' lifestyle and illustrations of their clothes, see De La Haye, Taylor, and Thompson (2005).
24. Mrs Cornwallis West was also instrumental in organizing the Shakespeare Ball in 1911 to raise funds for the new theatre at Stratford. On the early music revival, see Haskell (1988).
25. Later reconstructors of historical dances have contested these early attempts; see for example, Quirey and Holmes (1970).
26. *The Dance Journal,* March, p. 3.
27. *The Dance Journal,* May 1909, p. 1.

7   A Noble Profession

1. For an historical overview see the *International Encyclopedia of Dance* (1998). On French cultural leadership in dance see McGowan (2008) and on the Parisian dance scene, Cordova (1999). For more general cultural relations between London and Paris in the nineteenth century see Tombs and Tombs (2006).
2. A typical earlier example is that of Monsieur Rochefort, *Newcastle Courant,* 23 July 1831.
3. For examples, see Peel (1986); Thomas (1992); Flett and Flett (1964, 1979).
4. See, for example, Stewart (1938); also the late example in 1919, D'Egville (1937).
5. Young males and females from the gentry and upper-middle class were taught drill at some schools. Frances Power Cobbe (1894, vol. 1, p. 57) recalled a '"Capitaine" Somebody, who put us through manifold exercises with poles and dumbbells' at her school in Brighton during the 1830s. See also McIntosh (1968).
6. The claims date back at least to the Renaissance. See John Weaver (1712), his argument being much cited, often without credit, thereafter; see discussion in Ralph (1985).
7. Queen Victoria approved of this equipment, though Mme D'Egville Michau was against it. See Chapter 9.
8. Philip Richardson credits Mrs Wordsworth with the introduction of skipping and clubs into dancing class (*The Dancing Times,* July 1911, p. 242). Miss Leonora Geary's advertised use of clubs, however, in the 1840s makes this unlikely (*The Times,* 24 October 1843). Skipping-rope dances were a popular theatrical feature during the 1870s; see, for example, the painting *Harmony in Yellow and Gold. The Gold Girl* (1873) by James Whistler of child dancer Connie Gilchrist.
9. Langford (2000) provides an illuminating discussion on the deportment of the English as viewed by foreign eyes.
10. *The Book of Marie Taglioni. Little Anecdotes etc. Collected by Her Pupil Margaret Rolfe* unpublished diary (1885) and drawings are held in the Theatre and Performance Collections of the Victoria and Albert Museum, London. The files also contain later material contributed by the adult Rolfe. See Woodcock (1989). Subsequent reference to the collection here is by name alone.
11. See, for example, Stewart (1938); Asquith (1962); Asquith (1952).

12. See Cavers (1994), Buckland (2003), D'Egville (1937). For an obituary of Louis Hervet D'Egville senior, see *Dancing*, February 1892, p. 105. For that of his son see *The Dancing Times*, January 1928, pp. 534, 536, 545.
13. *The Dancing Times*, September 1919, p. 541.
14. July 1911 p. 242. See also, for example, Keppel (1958) and Asquith (1959).
15. See, for example, *The Times*, 10 August 1872, 24 January 1880, 3 May 1886, 1 November 1883, 18 September 1877.
16. *The Times*, 31 January 1872.
17. *The Times*, 15 November 1872.
18. Ibid. The Italian Opera was known as the Royal Opera House, Covent Garden from 1892.
19. *The Times*, 3 January 1872, 10 August 1872.
20. *The Times*, 7 December 1874. For further detail on the prestigious Espinosa family see Walker (2007).
21. *The Times*, 18 February 1876, 27 April 1882.
22. A guinea was worth twenty-one shillings (£1.05 in decimal currency). Comparing the purchasing power of money historically is by no means an exact science but for comparative present day values see www.nationalarchives. gov.uk/currency.
23. See, for example, *The Times*, 16 January 1873; Henderson [1879].
24. *The Dancing Times*, May 1898 and October 1899.
25. For Geary's *Companion to the Ball Room* see sixth edition in the library of Imperial Society of Teachers of Dancing, London; *The Times*, 31 January 1872, 16 January 1873; *The Times*, 7 December 1874. For Mr Bland's *Ball Room Companion, The Daily Telegraph*, 3 January 1870, 3 January 1872. For Henri Dacunha's pamphlet on dancing (1872) the Bodleian Library, Oxford. For Mrs Henderson's book [1850, third edition, 1852] and twentieth edition [1879], the British Library. For Humphrey [1874] the Bodleian Library, 1884 and 1889, the British Library. Lawson (1874) wrote an apologia for dance. For further accessible examples of dancing manuals see http://memory.loc. gov/ammem/dihtml/dihome.html (accessed 30 January 2011).
26. For *La Nationale* see LeBlanc [1883]; *The Hussars*, see *The Dancing Times*, May 1895, p. 4 and *The Era* 28 September 1895; for *Iolanthe*, see *Dancing*, June 1891 p. 4.
27. *The Dancing Times*, December 1924, p. 283.

8 Temples of Terpsichore

1. See, for example, *The Dancing Times*, March 1897, p. 8; *The Times*, 31 October 1890.
2. For theatrical connections of the Gilmer family, see *Dancing*, May 1892, p. 136; for the Souttens, see *The Dancing Times*, November 1913, pp. 85, 87.
3. On the system of articled pupils in music pedagogy see Ehrlich (1985); for examples in dance, see *The Times*, 24 February 1892, *The Dancing Times*, December 1897, p. 8.
4. See Census Returns 1901 and Buckland (2003).
5. *The Times*, 31 January 1872.
6. *The Times*, 24 November 1880, 23 September 1881.

7. See, for example, *The Times*, 10 March 1892; see Chapters 10, 11 and 12.
8. On advertising teacher and family connections see, for example, *The Times*, 22 February 1878, *The Times*, 27 February 1886, *Brighton Herald*, 30 May 1885. James Paul Michau, December 1883, London Probate Office. 'Contracts in Restraint of Trade', *The Dancing Times*, November, pp. 47, 49.
9. Edward Scott, Professor of Dancing and Physical Culture, advertisement in programme for *Monte Cristo, Jr.*, 25 July 1887, Theatre Royal and Opera House Brighton, p. 2. I am grateful to Jane Pritchard for this reference.
10. See *Dancing*, July 1891, p. 24; *The Dancing Times*, December 1897, p. 11.
11. This discussion owes much to Perkin (1989) and Thompson (1988). See, for example, Giovanni Vinio, Exeter Academy of Dancing, *The Period* 16 May 1891, reprinted *Dancing*, June 1891, pp. 6–7 and the ensuing correspondence.
12. See Buckland (2007). The *Dancing Times* alerted the capital's pedagogues to the annual call for applications and outcomes; see, for example, September 1894, October 1894, December 1894, May 1895, November 1896, October 1897.
13. For the case of Thomas Upton see *Dancing*, April 1893, p. 269; for the cases of Francis Piaggio and his appeal see *The Times*, 29 December, 1893, 2 February and 9 February, 9 April 1895.
14. See Buckland (2007); Edward Humphrey took care to note compliance with law and safety in his adverts.
15. See Isaac (1992); *The Dancing Times*, January 1914, p. 273.
16. The BATD regularly supplied a report of its annual convention for publication in the second series of *The Dancing Times*.
17. Husband and wife teams: Mr and Mrs Sheridan Lings taught in Holland Park, Notting Hill from the late 1870s (*The Times*, 7 February 1878); Mr and Mrs Jacques Wynman from Amsterdam were based in Newman Street, Oxford Street from the 1870s to the early 1890s (Census returns, 1871, 1881, advertisements in *The Times*). Here too was the academy of Mr and Mrs Nicholas Henderson, active as a partnership from the 1840s until her death in 1878. Mr Henderson continued teaching assisted by his daughter Elizabeth until his death in 1891. Dutchman Henri Dacunha was assisted by his two teenage daughters (1871 Census) in Soho Square; Bland by his daughters in Golden Square, St James and New Oxford Street; and Edouard LeBlanc advertised working with his daughters as assistants in Hart Street, Bloomsbury Square, *The Times*, 31 October 1877. It was not only men who were assisted by their daughters; see also Mme Isabel Bizet-Michau, *The Morning Post*, 1 October 1892.
18. *The Morning Post*, 6 February 1899; see also Chapter 10.
19. See for example, *The Times*, 14 January 1887 and the feature article on Miss Elizabeth Garratt (niece of Madame Stainton Taylor); 'The Dancing of the Day', *Pall Mall Gazette*, 14 April 1892.
20. See the recollections of De Valois (1957) and Bedells (1954). See also chapter 10.
21. *Hearth and Home*, 27 July reported in *The Dancing Times*, August 1911, p. 276.
22. *The Times* 13 November 1878; Tosh (1999).

9   The Fashioning of Ladies

1. For earlier perception of English typical character by foreigners see Langford (2000); Byron in *Don Juan* (1823) also refers to the 'serious Angles', canto xiv,

stanza 38. Numerous references to what were perceived as national characteristics of deportment and movement appear in dancing and etiquette
manuals, see also Grove (1895).

2. See, for example, 'The Drawing-Room, How Ladies are Trained for It', *Pall Mall Gazette*, 26 February 1889.
3. Opposition to female social dancing often dovetailed with puritanical and bourgeois condemnation of the lifestyle of the 'idle rich'. For a defence against religious condemnation see *The Dancing Times*, December 1896, pp. 2–3, p. 10, January 1897, pp. 1–3.
4. See, for example, *Punch*, 29 July 1871, 21 July 1877, 18 November 1899, Greville (1892).
5. 15 August 1891.
6. Candour, *The Daily Graphic*, 21 August 1891.
7. Detrimental, *The Daily Graphic*, 26 August 1891.
8. F.G.P., *The Morning Post*, 2 January 1899.
9. LADUD, *The Morning Post*, 17 January 1899.
10. *The Morning Post*, 17 January 1899.
11. Ibid.
12. *The Morning Post*, 20 January 1899.
13. *The Morning Post*, 17 December 1898.
14. *The Dancing Times*, December 1894, p. 7.
15. In Grove 1895, p. 416; Edward Lawson, *The Morning Post*, 4 January 1899.
16. Not an "Up to Date" Young Woman, *The Daily Graphic*, 18 August 1891.
17. Freelance quoted in An Old Fashioned Man, *The Daily Graphic*, 28 August 1891.
18. Up to Date, *The Daily Graphic*, 28 September 1891.
19. See, for example, W. Hill, *The Morning Post*, 23 January 1899.
20. 12 April; see also *Dancing*, December 1891, p. 83 and Chapter 10.

10 Modelling the Lady

1. *The Queen* quoted in *Dancing*, July 1891, p. 21.
2. *The Times*, 24 December 1898.
3. Her marriage to Frederick Wellesley was short lived (*ODNB*). John Ruskin and Sir Edward Burne-Jones were fervent admirers (Flitch, 1912). The Countess of Russell and her sister reputedly legitimated the dance for Society by their performances at a charity matinée in a London theatre (Flitch, 1912).
4. *Dancing*, July 1891, p. 21.
5. *Dancing*, July 1891, p. 21. Consuelo Vanderbilt recalled how Margot Asquith performed skirt dances in later life 'delighting to prove the suppleness of her sixty years' (Balsan, 1953, p. 165).
6. See Grossmith (in Naylor, 1913); Nevill (1912); Jupp (1923); Macqueen-Pope (1949, 1956); Bingham (1980); Hyman (1975); Bailey (1996).
7. *Pall Mall Gazette*, 4 June 1890; 14 April 1892; *Dancing*, June 1891, p. 3; Malcolm (1932).
8. On the appearance of theatrical people at Society events see, for example, Armytage (1927). *The Times*, 23 September 1908 (Mabel, Lady Russell); Richardson (1913).
9. *Pall Mall Gazette*, 14 April 1892.

11   Where Are Our Men?

1. The letters written in 1783 have had a long and complex history of reproduction. See entries in British Library catalogue.
2. Anon. [1878], p. 115. This requirement is evident as far back as Castiglione's *Il Cortegiano* of 1528; see McGowan (2008).
3. See also Chapter 16. For discussion of the French dancing master as a figure of ridicule see Leppert (1988). The idea of 'pitying superiority' of the English towards the 'French dancing-master' prevailed, see Grove (1895), p. 124.
4. Even the celebrated Michau family during the 1830s ran the risk of social exclusion from Society balls, see *The Times*, 29 February 1836.
5. *Pall Mall Gazette*, 24 February 1888; on late Victorian male evening dress, see Cunnington and Cunnington (1966).
6. 'An Old Fogey', *The Daily Graphic*, 25 September 1891; 'Up to Date' countered that dancing 'as a means of exercise … is far inferior to lawn tennis', *The Daily Graphic*, 28 September 1891.
7. See, for example, 'White Lies', *Punch*, 9 July 1892.
8. *Judy*, 26 December 1883.
9. *The Idler* quoted in *Dancing*, February 1893, p. 245; see also the ironically labelled cartoon, 'Dancing Men', *Punch*, 12 March 1892.
10. Williams (1892), p. 371; see too Crompton's editorial in *Dancing*, January 1893.
11. *Punch*, 20 September 1890.
12. 'Is Dancing Degenerating?', *The Dance Journal*, July 1908, p. 8.
13. See, for example, F.G.P., *The Morning Post*, 2 January 1899; A Primrose Dame, *The Morning Post*, 23 January 1899.

12   Dancing Dogs and Manly Men

1. Pas de Quatre, *Dancing*, March 1893, p. 262. Alexandra's partners were Oliver Montagu, Arthur Paget, Gerald Paget, Augustus Lumley and Harry Chaplin.
2. See, for example, 'Dancing Men', (du Maurier, 1897), *Punch*, 1 April 1882.
3. *The Daily News*, 28 March 1884.
4. *Sala's Journal* quoted in *Dancing*, March 1893, p. 261. See also *Moonshine*, 28 December 1889, *Punch*, 6 May 1882, *Punch*, 6 July 1889 and du Maurier (1897).
5. On their growing scarcity see, for example, *Judy*, 26 August 1891, *Fun*, 31 March 1896.
6. Dancing was taught in numerous boys' schools in the eighteenth century. See *Gentleman's Magazine* 1736 quoted in Leppert (1988, p. 81), with respect to the absence of dance tuition at Eton and Cambridge. Presumably Esher (Eton and Cambridge) and Cornwallis West (Eton and Sandhurst) took (or retained proficiency from) private lessons. Adverts from the 1840s in *The Times* for boys' schools which specifically include dancing relate to 'Education Francaise for Young Gentlemen'. See 26 September 1843. For children's gendered attitudes towards dancing see, for example, *Punch*, 24 February 1872.
7. See Crompton's editorial, *Dancing*, July 1891, p. 15.

8. On repaying hospitality see, for example, 'A Slave to Courtesy', *Punch*, 22 July 1893.
9. 26 August. Letter signed 'Detrimental. Bachelors' Club'.
10. Association v. Rugby, *Punch*, 18 December 1894; *Punch*, 25 May 1872.
11. *Dancing*, December 1891, p. 81. The soubriquet reputedly derives from their refusal to dance when stationed at Dublin earlier in the nineteenth century; Richardson thought it untrue of their later practice, *The Dancing Times*, July 1912, p. 371. On military deportment and dancing see 'Modern Types. The Young Guardsman', 'his nationality and his profession both forbid him to display an excess of enthusiasm', *Punch*, 10 May 1890 and Scott (1887a). Female members of military families also adopted the bearing, see Duncan (1891).
12. *Dancing Times*, April 1913, p. 416.
13. *Dancing*, December 1891, p. 81.
14. *Dancing*, January 1892, p. 94.
15. *Punch*, 17 April 1858.
16. *The Dancing Times*, November, p. 5.
17. *Dancing*, January 1893, p. 231.
18. *The Morning Post*, 17 January 1899, p. 3.
19. W.P., *Dancing*, March 1893, p 262.
20. Billy, *Dancing*, March 1893, p. 262.
21. Popular British patriotism attributed Winston Churchill with the tenacity and strength of the British bulldog; a typical aristocrat of his period, he always preferred poodles.

13 Moving into the Twentieth Century

1. See, for example, 'Manners and Modes. A Young Girl has the Temerity to Bring a Chaperon to a Dance.' *Punch*, 25 February 1920. For a personal aristocratic male perspective on changes in the new century see Malcolm (1932).
2. *The Dancing Times*, October, 1910, p. 12.
3. *The Dancing Times*, October 1912, p. 17; see also the clubs listed in the monthly 'Dancing News' of *The Dancing Times*.
4. *The Dancing Times*, October, 1910, p. 9, October 1912, p. 17. For more detail on the Empress Rooms see *The Dancing Times*, November 1912, p. 93. See also, Our London Ball Rooms, *The Dancing Times*, October 1913, p. 10.
5. See for example, *The Dancing Times*, September 1911, p. 287.
6. For examples of notations and specialist discussion of the Boston see, for example, Sheafe (1913) and Scott (1913).
7. See opinions in 'Will the Boston Live?', *The Dancing Times*, October 1910, pp. 9–10 and November, 1910, pp. 33–4. There was considerable confusion on the part of those unfamiliar with the Boston, many of whom wrongly bracketed it with the new ragtime dances and the Tango: see, for example, *The Daily Telegraph*, February 1913 and *The Times*, May 1913 correspondence. On musical accompaniment, see 'The Rise of English Waltz Composers', *The Dancing Times*, November 1910, pp. 34–5.
8. The Boston, The Double Boston, *The Dance Journal*, January 1913, pp. 2–5; *The Dancing Times*, August 1913, p. 700.

14 Modernizing Terpsichore

1. See Carter (2005b); 'For some time past, there has been a rage for stage dancing at the London music-halls,' *The Morning Post*, 20 April, 1910. On musical theatre of the period, see Macqueen-Pope (1956), Seeley and Bunnett (1989) and Platt (2004).
2. There were numerous guide books to Parisian entertainment for foreigners, see, for example, Richardson [1910]. See also Hindson (2007).
3. See Kift (1996), Donohue (2005), Bailey (1986 and 2003) and Clayton (2005).
4. See, for example, the coverage of Anna Pavlova, Tamara Karsavina and Irene Castle in *The Tatler* and *The Daily Sketch*.
5. See 'A Plea for Greater Variety in the Ballroom', *Punch*, 13 April, 1910 which lampoons music-hall dance acts.
6. On blacking-up in Britain, see Pickering (2008); on *In Dahomey* in Britain see *The Era*, 23 May 1903; see also Parsonage (2005).
7. *The Penny Illustrated Paper*, 6 April 1907; Macqueen-Pope (1956). For a romanticized account of how the Apache came to the Parisian stage see Mouvet [1915].
8. *The Dance Journal*, May 1911, p. 5.
9. For accounts of the Castles' careers see Golden (2007) and Castle (1919, 1958). See also Cook (1999).
10. *The Dancing Times*, December 1913, p. 132. He made a favourable comparison with Marquis with respect to upper body carriage and earlier had recommended male readers to study Oscar's dancing as a model; see Oscar and Suzette, 'A Study in Perfect Carriage', *The Dancing Times*, March 1912, pp. 168, 169 and April 1914, p. 425.
11. Oscar appeared first in London with Regine as partner in the previous autumn, see *The Times*, 25 September 1911 and *The Times*, 26 October 1911 when their dancing was noted as being 'practical for the ballroom and full of grace'; 'Star Turns. The Perfect Dancers: Oscar and Suzette', *The Sketch*, 21 February 1912.
12. 20 January. See Chapter 16.
13. Several West End female teachers did offer ballet as adverts and features in *The Dancing Times* testify.
14. *The Dancing Times*, November 1910, p. 33, December 1911, p. 7. See Chapter 15.
15. *The Dancing Times*, December 1913, p. 132.
16. *The Dancing Times*, December 1913, p. 171. The craze was satirized in the song 'Tommy, Won't You Teach Me How to Tango' (1913) performed by George Grossmith Junior.
17. See, in particular, 'Tango Teas. By One Who Goes to Them', *The Dancing Times*, December 1913, pp. 134–36, as well as the numerous adverts in *The Dancing Times*, national and local newspapers.
18. *Dancing*, September 1892, pp. 190–1.
19. *The Dancing Times*, October 1913, p. 13.
20. *The Dancing Times*, December 1915, p. 81.
21. See the numerous adverts in *The Dancing Times* especially from October 1913 onwards.
22. 'What To Do With Our Girls', *The Dancing Times*, August 1914, p. 689.

23. See *The Dancing Times*, June 1914 pp. 562–3, July 1914, p. 616; for war-time activities see, for example, *The Dancing Times*, November 1914, p. 46, January 1916, pp. 130, 138 and Chapter 15.

15 Civilization Under Threat

1. *Punch* satirized this drive for exotic novelty dancing by depicting a music-hall entrepreneur auditioning at the North Pole, 16 August 1911.
2. Although dealing primarily with a slightly later period, see Robinson (2006) and Gottschild (2002) on the white exclusivity of the profession.
3. See, for example, *Dancing Times*, December 1913, p. 132.
4. See 'Terpsichorean Terrors' [Maurice and Florence Walton], *The Tatler*, 27 March 1912; Oscar and Suzette in a crouching pose in *The Tatler*, 21 February 1912, 4 September 1912, 18 December 1912; for a defence of the dance see Hewitt (1912).
5. Hints to Climbers: How to Attract Notice, *Punch*, 11 June 1913.
6. See, for example, *Punch*, 7 February 1912, 14 February 1912.
7. See, for example, 'For Ball-Room Use? The Extra!', *The Sketch*, May 1912, p. 124.
8. The *Dancing Times* first published, with Walter Humphrey's help, 'How to Dance The Tango', with illustrations of Mons. Robert in February 1911, pp. 106–7. See also *The Dancing Times*, September 1911, p. 290, July 1913, p. 655 and 'Where To Learn the Tango', *The Dancing Times*, October 1913, pp. 19–20, 23, 25.
9. Richardson thought Almanos and Odette the best Tango dancers of all (1946); see also *The Dancing Times*, November 1913, p. 67. 'Tango Teas. By One Who Goes To Them', *The Dancing Times*, December 1913, pp. 134–6; Marquis and Miss Clayton [1913] demonstrated the Tango on roller skates at the Earl's Court rink, see *The Dancing Times*, December 1913, p. 132.
10. George Grossmith Junior reckoned himself among the first to move onto the floor in London (Richardson, 1946). For a list of clubs see, for example, 'The Leading London Dance Clubs', *The Dancing Times*, November 1913, pp. 75–7, December 1913, pp. 167, 169.
11. *The Sketch*, 3 April 1912; see too *The Sketch*, 14 August 1912 (Maurice and Florence Walton); for other exhibition Tango images see, for example, *The Dancing Times*, January 1913, p. 239 (M. Robert and Mlle Gaby), May 1913, pp. 480, 481 (Maurice and Florence Walton); December 1913 cover (M. Marquis and Miss Clayton); January 1914, p. 227 (Roland and Marion Mitford).
12. 'The Truth At Last', *The Dancing Times*, July 1914, pp. 606–7.
13. *The Dancing Times*, August 1914, p. 664.
14. *The Dancing Times*, September 1914, p. 715.
15. *The Dancing Times*, December 1914, p. 115.
16. For experiences of and responses to dancing in wartime London see, for example, *The Times* reports and correspondence: 21 December 1914, 10 March 1915, 6 December 1916, 2 March 1917, 26 October 1918. 'For a short while men and women sought to forget war during the brief second or two in the lilt of a valse, and made themselves drunk with dancing'

(X, Countess of, 1932, p. 119); *The Dancing Times* continued its monthly reports throughout, including those of fatalities from the dance world from November 1914.

17. For an overview of the early days of the Foxtrot in England, see Richardson (1946) and 'A Fox Trot Symposium', *The Dancing Times*, June 1915, pp. 307–11.

18. Silvester and Richardson (1936); during part of the war, Belle Harding was assisted by Mons. Pierre who was unable to enlist because of poor eyesight.

19. *The Dancing Times*, April 1947, p. 365.

20. See, for example, 'Miss Phyllis Monkman and "The Saunter"', *The Dancing Times*, October 1916, pp. 13, 15.

16 Knuts and Aliens

1. On the distinction between a 'blood' and a 'nut', see Grossmith in Naylor (1913), especially the accompanying plates in which the embodied class ideal of the English gentleman is finely depicted in dress and posture.

2. On dinner jackets and the shift towards informality in male dress, especially through the rise of leisure activities such as golf and motoring, see Mansfield and Cunnington (1973), Breward (1999), Nevill (1912) and Malcolm (1932).

3. *The Times*, 20 May and 21 May 1913; 'Dancing Notes', *Punch's Almanack for 1914*.

4. It is likely that the Boston was a contributory factor to Oxford and Cambridge male students' interest in attending dance classes from 1905, see *The Dancing Times*, May 1911, p. 189.

5. *The Dancing Times*, January 1914, p. 304.

6. H. R. Wakefield, 'Reply to a "Peeress"', *The Times*, 21 May 1913.

7. On the Victorian versus modern girl in the ballroom see, for example, letter from Percy Moenich, *The Times*, 24 May 1913 and A Girl Who Dances, *The Times*, 23 May 1913.

8. 'Introductions at Dances', *The Times*, 20 May 1914. 'The Day of Youthful Grandmothers', *The Times*, 14 May 1914.

9. Quoted in *The Dancing Times*, January 1911, p. 90. On female fashion of the period see Mansfield and Cunnington (1973).

10. On Poiret, see Koda and Bolton (2007); on Lucile, see Mendes and De La Haye (2009); *Punch*, 23 July 1913.

11. 20 May. Correspondence poured in over the next few weeks and was reflected elsewhere in national, local and specialist press. For George Grossmith Junior's reflections on the controversy and the Tango see Naylor (1913).

12. H. R. Wakefield, *The Times*, 21 May 1913.

13. *The Daily Star*, 10 February 1912.

14. May 1911, p. 10; October 1910, p. 10.

15. 7 February 1912.

16. Ibid.

17. 23 May 1913.

18. See, in particular, Wagner (1997), Cook (1997), Robinson (2004) and George-Graves (2009).
19. Though social and racial barriers were still extensive, of course, in the USA; see Robinson (2009).
20. The earlier humane sentiment that had fed the abolition of slavery in 1833 had largely given way to resurgence of antagonistic racism in the wake of the Morant Bay Rebellion on Jamaica in 1865. Eminent Victorian writers Thomas Carlyle and Anthony Trollope expanded upon virulent anti-black feeling articulated by eighteenth-century writers, notably philosopher David Hume who asserted in 1771 that there 'never was a civilized nation of any other complexion than white' and Edward Long whose bigoted views as a member of the Caribbean planter elite with direct experience of black people, carried especial weight. See Hall (2000a).
21. 'Modern Dancing. A Controversy and a Retrospect. The Need for Beau Nash', *The Times*, 23 May 1913; Hyatt-Woolf (1911, p.5).
22. *The Saturday Review*, 24 May 1913; see Cecil Taylor, *The Times*, 23 May 1913, Oscar Browning, *The Times*, 2 June 1913.
23. *ODNB*; *Punch*, 9 April 1913.
24. On religious and moral opposition to the theatre see Foulkes (1997) and Donohue (2005).
25. H. R. Wakefield, *The Times*, 21 May 1913.
26. *The Times*, 23 May 1913.
27. 'Bohemia in Mayfair. A Dance, Some Dancers and a Moral', *The Dance Journal* 1910, p. 13.
28. Scott's first letter was published 3 February 1913 in *The Daily Telegraph* and provoked numerous responses in the following week (his last letter appeared 10 February.) Crompton was similarly opposed to the new dances, see *The Daily Express*, 19 February 1912.
29. 'Manner in Social Dancing', *The Dancing Times*, December 1917, pp. 63–67; *Brighton Herald*, 22 March 1912.
30. *The Times*, 24 May 1913.
31. *Brighton Herald*, 24 October 1914. See also D'Egville in *The Dancing Times*, August 1919, p. 45.
32. *The Dance Journal*, 1910, p. 13.

17   Civilizing from the Centre

1. See Buckland (2007); *The Dancing Times*, November 1914, p. 54; http://www.ukadance.co.uk accessed 29 September 2010; *The Dancing Times*, May 1914, p. 525. See also *The Dancing Times*, February 1917, pp. 156–57, 173.
2. For a brief early history of the ballroom branch see Richardson (1946).
3. *The Dancing Times*, August 1913, pp. 697–9, October 1913, p. 27; compare Crompton's similar difficulties two decades earlier (Buckland, 2007).
4. By 1914 Mrs H. R. Johnson had become a Vice-President of the BATD (*The Dancing Times*, September 1914, p. 725); by 1924 the ISDT had established its genre-specific branches, see ISTD (2004).
5. *Dancing*, July 1891, p. 16; *The Dancing Times*, December 1915, p. 113.

6. *The Dancing Times*, May 1911, p. 202.
7. *The Dancing Times*, July 1911, p. 250.
8. *The Dancing Times*, March 1911, p. 154; *The Dancing Times*, October 1913, p. 17; *The Dancing Times*, April 1915, p. 263.
9. See, for example, Golden (2007) and Cook (1998); *The Dancing Times*, July 1914, pp. 607–8.
10. The 'Sitter Out' was also a regular feature in the first series of *The Dancing Times*. See entry on Richardson in *ODNB*.
11. *The Dancing Times*, February 1919, p. 152, February 1918, pp. 152–3; Richardson (1946).
12. *Punch*, 22 January 1919, p. 69.
13. *The Dancing Times*, January 1918, p. 128.
14. *The Dancing Times*, October 1919, p. 2.
15. *The Dancing Times*, July 1914, p. 634.
16. *The Dancing Times*, November 1918, p. 34.
17. *The Dancing Times*, January 1914, p. 304.
18. It is noteworthy that as a result of the early high death rate of upper-class males at the front, a number of men from lower down the social scale were elevated to the officer class and sought to retain their new status and manner in post-war Britain. See James (2006, p. 412) on 'temporary gentlemen'. Such apparent genteel behaviour from lower-middle and upper working-class dancers has been critiqued as affectation, see Fiske and Hartley (1993) and the ethnographic rejoinder from Penny (1999). See Carden-Coyne (2009) on cultural responses to the impact of the First World War in moves to re-build civilization through the site of the human body.
19. *The Daily Sketch*, 11 October.
20. *The Dancing Times*, October 1919, p. 3; on dance bands see Parsonage (2005) and Nott (2002).
21. 12 May 1920.
22. *The Dancing Times*, April 1920, pp. 526, 528, May 1920, p. 606. Maurice Mouvet was generally known simply as Maurice in Britain and, in the early days of his career, by his American name of Morris in continental Europe, thus capitalising on the cachet of exotic authentic 'other' in each instance.
23. *The Dancing Times*, June 1920, pp. 686–90, 692, 697, 699, 701, 703, 705, 707. See Cresswell (2006) for an interpretation of the standardization as a mode of mobility.
24. This view of the Ballets Russes' influence and standing has been re-appraised from alternative perspectives: see, for example, Carter (2005a) and Järvinen (2008).
25. *The Dancing Times*, May 1920, p. 606.
26. The point is similarly made by Colls (2002). More generally on the notion of Englishness, see Mandler (2006).
27. *The Dancing Times*, June 1920, p. 703.
28. See, for example, 'Get the London Style', *The Dancing Times*, February 1922, pp. 424–8, 'Ballroom Dancing in France. "English Style" Finds Favour', *The Dancing Times*, March 1928, pp. 829–33; Bradley (1947); Silvester (1958).

18   Looking Back, Moving On

1. *The Dance Journal*, March 1909, p. 12.
2. Whereas the folk dance revival has received considerable attention, see, for example, Boyes (1993) and Gammon (2008), the historical dance movement in Britain awaits critical scrutiny.
3. All these dances first appeared in America. The Kensington Crawl was considered by both Grossmith and Scott as an American variant of the Waltz.
4. The notion of 'scape' owes much to Appadurai (1996) and Slobin (1993).

Bibliography

A Member of the Aristocracy (1879). *Manners and Tone of Good Society*. London: Frederick Warne Co. revised editions 1888, 1910.

Abra, A. J. (2009). *On with the Dance: Nation, Culture, and Popular Dancing in Britain, 1918–1945*. PhD dissertation, University of Michigan.

Adams, J. E. (1995). *Dandies and Desert Saints. Styles of Victorian Masculinity*. Ithaca and London: Cornell University Press.

Adshead-Lansdale, J. and Layson, J. (eds) (1994). *Dance History: An Introduction*. 2nd edn. London and New York: Routledge.

Albright, A. C. (2003/2004). 'Matters of Tact: Writing History from the Inside Out', *Dance Research Journal*, 35, 2 and 36, 1, 11–26.

Aldrich, E. (1990). 'A New Look at an Old Dance: The Waltz', *5th Hong Kong International Dance Conference Proceedings*, vol. 1, 29–46.

——— (1991). *From the Ballroom to Hell. Grace and Folly in Nineteenth-Century Dance*. Evanston, Illinois: Northwestern University Press.

——— (2005). *An American Ballroom Companion. Dance Instruction Manuals ca. 1490–1920*, for the Music Division, Library of Congress, http://memory.loc.gov/ammem/dihtml/dihome.html accessed 31 January 2011.

——— (2009). 'The Civilizing of America's Ballrooms' in J. Malnig (2009b).

Allen, D. and Jordan, S. (eds) (1993). *Parallel Lines: Media Representations of Dance*. London: John Libby.

Altick, R. D. (1957). *The English Common Reader: A Social History of the Mass Reading Public, 1800–1900*. Chicago and London: University of Chicago Press.

Ancaster, Countess (1895). 'Balls: Hostesses and Guests'. In L. Grove.

Anon. [1874]. *The Ball-Room Guide. A Handy Manual for All Classes of Society. With Costumes for Fancy and Calico Balls*. London: F. Warne & Co.

Anon. [1878]. *Etiquette for Ladies and Gentlemen or, Principles of True Politeness*. London: Milner & Co.

Appadurai, A. (1996). *Modernity at Large. Cultural Dimensions of Globalization*. Minneapolis, MN: University of Minnesota Press.

Armstrong, L. H. [1900]. *The Ball-Room Guide*. London and New York: Frederick Warne & Co.

Armytage, Hon. Mrs (1883). *Old Court Customs and Modern Court Rule*. London: Richard Bentley & Son.

Armytage, P. (1927). *By the Clock of St. James's*. London: John Murray.

Asquith, C. (1952). *Remember and Be Glad*. London: James Barrie.

——— (1950). *Haply I May Remember*. London: James Barrie.

Asquith, M. A. E. (1962). *The Autobiography of Margot Asquith*. Edited by M. Bonham Carter. London: Eyre & Spottiswoode.

Baedeker, C. (1908). *London and Its Environs*. 3rd edn. Leipzig: Karl Baedeker.

Bailey, P. (1986). *Music Hall. The Business of Pleasure*. Milton Keynes: Open University Press.

——— (1996). '"Naughty but Nice": Musical Comedy and the Rhetoric of the Girl, 1892–1914'. In J. H. Kaplan and M. R. Booth.

—— (2003). *Popular Culture and Performance in the Victorian City*. Cambridge: Cambridge University Press.

Balsan, C. V. (1953). *The Glitter and the Gold*. Melbourne, London and Toronto: William Heinemann.

Banes, S. (1998). *Dancing Women. Female Bodies on Stage*. London: Routledge.

Barkin, E. and Hamessley, L. (eds) (1999). *Audible Traces: Gender, Identity and Music*. Zürich: Carcifoli Verlagshaus.

Barnes, H. (1908). 'A Glimpse at the London Music Halls. The Typical Amusement Resorts of the British Metropolis', *Munsey's Magazine*.

Beckett, J. V. (1986). *The Aristocracy in England 1660–1914*. New York: Basil Blackwell.

Bedells, P. (1954). *My Dancing Days*. London: Phoenix House.

Berlin, E. A. (1980). *Ragtime. A Musical and Cultural History*. Berkeley, Los Angeles and London: University of California Press.

Bingham, M. (1980). *Earls and Girls. Dramas in High Society*. London: Hamish Hamilton.

Bourdieu, P. (1984). *Distinction: A Social Critique of the Judgement of Taste*, trans. R. Nice. Cambridge, Mass: Harvard University Press.

Boyle, C. (1873). 'Ball-Giving and Ball-Going', *Macmillan's Magazine*, 27, 458–68.

Boyes, G. (1993). *The Imagined Village. Culture, Ideology and the English Folk Revival*. Manchester: Manchester University Press.

Bradley, J. (1947). *Dancing Through Life*. London: Hollis & Carter.

Brake, L. (2001). *Print in Transition, 1850–1910*. Basingstoke: Palgrave Macmillan.

Bratton, J. S. (1990). 'Dancing a Hornpipe in Fetters', *Folk Music Journal*, 6, no. 1, 65–82.

Breward, C. (1999). *The Hidden Consumer. Masculinities, Fashion, and City Life, 1860–1914*. Manchester: Manchester University Press.

Brooks, L. M. (2002). 'Dance History and Method: A Return to Meaning', *Dance Research*, 20, no. 1, 33–53.

Brown, L. (1985). *Victorian News and Newspapers*. Oxford: Clarendon Press.

Bryant, M. (2000). *Dictionary of Twentieth-Century British Cartoonists and Caricaturists*. Aldershot: Ashgate.

Bryson, N. (1997). 'Cultural Studies and Dance History'. In J. C. Desmond (ed.).

Buckland, T. J. (2003). 'Edward Scott: The Last of the English Dancing Masters', *Dance Research*, 21, 2, 3–35.

—— (2006). *Dancing from Past to Present. Nation, Culture, Identities*. Madison, WI: University of Wisconsin Press.

—— (2007).'Crompton's Campaign: The Professionalisation of Dance Pedagogy in Late Victorian England', *Dance Research*, 25, 1, 1–34.

Buckley, R. R. (1911). *The Shakespeare Revival and the Stratford-upon-Avon Movement*. London: George Allen & Sons.

Buckman, P. (1978). *Let's Dance. Social, Ballroom and Folk Dancing*. New York and London: Paddington Press.

Bush, M. L. (1984). *The English Aristocracy*. Manchester: Manchester University Press.

Burke, P. (2004). *What is Cultural History?* Cambridge: Polity.

Burt, R. (2007). *The Male Dancer. Bodies, Spectacle, Sexualities*. 2nd edn. London: Routledge.

Caffyn, J. (1998). *Sussex Schools in the 18ᵗʰ Century. Schooling, Provision, Schoolteachers and Scholars*. Lewes: Sussex Record Society.

Carden-Coyne, A. (2009). *Reconstructing the Body: Classicism, Modernism and the First World War*. Oxford and New York: Oxford University Press.

Campbell, C., Lady. (1893). *Etiquette of Good Society*. Edited and revised by Lady C. Campbell. London: Cassell & Co.

Cannadine, D. (1996). *The Decline and Fall of the British Aristocracy*. London: Papermac.

—— (ed.) (2002). *What Is History Now?* Basingstoke: Palgrave Macmillan.

Carter, A. (2004a). 'Destabilising the Discipline: Critical Debates About History and Their Impact on the Study of Dance'. In A. Carter (ed.).

—— (ed.) (2004b). *Rethinking Dance History: A Reader*. London and New York: Routledge.

—— (2005a). *Dance and Dancers in the Victorian and Edwardian Music Hall Ballet*. Aldershot, Hampshire: Ashgate.

—— (2005b). 'London, 1908: A Synchronic View of History', *Dance Research*, 23, 1, 36–50.

Cassells. [c.1880]. *Cassells Household Guide*, 4 vols. London: Cassell, Petter & Galpin.

Castle, I. (1919). *My Husband*. London: John Lane.

—— (1958). *Castles in the Air*. Garden City, New York: Doubleday.

Castle, V. and Castle, I. (1914). *Modern Dancing*. London and New York: Harper & Bros.

Cavers, K. (1994). 'Some Talk of Alexander'. James Harvey D'Egville and the 'English' Ballet 1770–1836. Unpublished MPhil thesis, University of Surrey.

Chamberlin, J. E. and Gilman, S. L. (1985). *Degeneration: The Dark Side of Progress*. New York: Columbia University Press.

Chancellor, E. B. (1908). *The Private Palaces of London Past and Present*. London: Kegan Paul, Trench, Trübner & Co.

Chaplin, N. (1911). *Court Dances and Others. Revived by N. Chaplin*. London: J. Curwen & Sons.

Clayton, A. (2005). *Decadent London. Fin de Siècle City*. London: Historical Publications.

Cobbe, F. P. (1894). *Life of Francis Power Cobbe, by Herself*. Boston and New York: Houghton Mifflin.

Cohen, M. (1996). *Fashioning Masculinity. National Identity and Language in the Eighteenth Century*. London and New York: Routledge.

—— (2005). '"Manners" Make the Man: Politeness, Chivalry, and the Construction of Masculinity, 1750–1830', *Journal of British Studies*, 44, 2, 312–29.

Cohen, S. R. (2000). *Art, Dance, and the Body in French Culture of the Ancien Régime*. Cambridge: Cambridge University Press.

Coles, A. M. C. [1909]. *Old English Country Dance Steps*. London: J. Curwen & Sons.

—— (1910). *The Hornpipe. The Steps Recorded by Miss A. M. C. Coles*. London: J. Curwen & Sons.

Colley, L. (2005). *Britons. Forging the Nation 1707–1837*. 2nd edn. New Haven and London: Yale University Press.

Collier, S., Cooper, A., Azzi, A. S. and Martin, R. (1995). *Tango: The Dance, the Song, the Story*. London: Thames & Hudson.

Colls, R. (2002). *Identity of England*. Oxford: Oxford University Press.

Constantine, S., Kirby M. W. and Rose, M. B. (eds) (1995). *The First World War in British History*. London: Edward Arnold.

Contributors, Twenty-Seven (1932). *Fifty Years. Memories and Contrasts. A Composite Picture of the Period 1882–1932*. London: Thornton Butterworth.

Cook, S. C. (1997). 'Tango Lizards and Girlish Men: Performing Masculinity on the Social Dance Floor', *Proceedings of the 20th Society of Dance History Scholars Conference*, Barnard College, New York City, 41–53.

——— (1998). 'Passionless Dancing and Passionate Reform: Respectability, Modernism, and the Social Dancing of Irene and Vernon Castle'. In W. Washabaugh.

——— (1999). 'Watching our Step: Embodying Research, Telling Stories'. In E. Barkin and L. Hamessley (eds).

Cooper, A. (1995). 'Tangomania in Europe and North America 1913–1914'. In Collier et al.

Cooper, D. (1958). *The Rainbow Comes and Goes*. London: Rupert Hart-Davies.

Cordova, S. D. (1999). *Paris Dances: Textual Choreographies in the Nineteenth-Century French Novel*. San Francisco; London: International Scholars Publications.

Cowles, V. (1956). *Edward VII and His Circle*. London: Hamish Hamilton.

Cresswell, T. (2006). '"You Cannot Shake that Shimmie Here": Producing Mobility on the Dance Floor', *Cultural Geographies*, 13, 55–77.

Crompton, R. M. [1891]. *Theory and Practice of Modern Dancing*. London: Willcocks & Co.

Crook, J. M. (1999). *The Rise of the Nouveaux Riches. Style and Status in Victorian and Edwardian Architecture*. London: John Murray.

Crow, D. (1971). *The Victorian Woman*. London: Allen & Unwin.

Crozier, G. B. [1913]. *The Tango and How to Dance It*. London: Andrew Melrose.

Cunnington, C. W. and Cunnington, P. (1966). *Handbook of English Costume in the Nineteenth Century*. London: Faber and Faber.

Dacunha, H. (1872). *The Companion to the Ball Room and Self-Instructor in the Art of Dancing, Etiquette, etc.* London (copy in Bodleian Library).

Daunton, M. J. and Rieger, B. (eds) (2001). *Meanings of Modernity. Britain from the Late-Victorian Era to World War II*. Oxford: Berg.

Davidoff, L. (1973). *The Best Circles. Society Etiquette and the Season*. London: Croom Helm.

Davis, T. C. (1991). *Actresses as Working Women. Their Social Identity in Victorian Culture*. London and New York: Routledge.

D'Egville, A. (1937). *Adventures in Safety*. London: Sampson, Low, Marston.

D'Egville, L. (1917). 'Manner (Deportment) and Dancing', *The Dancing Times*, September, p. 356.

D'Egville Michau, Mme C. (1861). *Treatise on Deportment, Dancing and Physical Education for Young Ladies*. London: T.C. Newby.

De Grazia, V. with Furlough, E. (ed.) (1996). *The Sex of Things. Gender and Consumption in Historical Perspective*. Berkley and Los Angeles, California: University of California Press.

Dickens, C. (1853). *Bleak House*. London: Bradbury and Evans.

De La Haye, A., Taylor, L. and Thompson, E. (2005). *A Family of Fashion. The Messels: Six Generations of Dress*. London: Philip Wilson.

Delamont, S. and Duffin, L. (1978). *The Nineteenth-Century Woman. Her Cultural and Physical World*. London: Croom Helm.

De Valois, N. (1957). *Come Dance with Me: A Memoir 1898–1956*. London: Hamish Hamilton.

Desmond, J. C. (ed.). (1997). *Meaning in Motion: New Cultural Studies of Dance* Durham: Duke University Press.

Dils, A. and Albright, A. C. (eds). (2001). *Moving History/Dancing Cultures: A Dance History Reader*. Middletown, Conn.: Wesleyan University Press.

Donohue, J. (2005). *Fantasies of Empire. The Empire Theatre of Varieties, Leicester Square, and the Licensing Controversy of 1894*. Iowa City: University of Iowa Press.

Duffin, L. (1978). 'Prisoners of Progress: Women and Evolution' in Delamont and Duffin (1978).

Du Maurier, G. (1897). *English Society*. New York: Harper & Bros.

Duncan, S. J. (1891). *An American Girl in London*. London: Chatto & Windus.

Dyer, R. (1997). *White*. London: Routledge.

Dyhouse, C. (1976). 'Social Darwinistic Ideas and the Development of Women's Education in England, 1880–1920', *History of Education*, 5, no. 1, 41–58.

Ehrlich, C. (1985). *The Music Profession in Britain since the Eighteenth Century: A Social History*. Oxford: Clarendon Press.

Elias, N. (1978). *The Civilising Process: Vol.1, The History of Manners*. New York: Pantheon Books.

Eliot, George. (1876). *Daniel Deronda*. Edinburgh and London: William Blackwood & Sons.

Engelhardt, M. (2009). *Dancing Out of Line. Ballrooms, Ballets, and Mobility in Victorian Fiction and Culture*. Athens, Ohio: Ohio University Press.

Engen, R. K. (1991). *Sir John Tenniel: Alice's White Knight*. Aldershot: Scolar Press.

Erenberg, L. A. (1981). *Steppin' Out. New York Nightlife and the Transformation of American Culture 1890–1930*. Chicago: University of Chicago Press.

Esher, R. B. B. (1927). *Cloud-Capp'd Towers*. London: John Murray.

Evans, H. and Evans, M. (1976). *The Party that Lasted 100 Days. The Late Victorian Season: A Social Study*. London: MacDonald and Jane's.

Farnell, B. (1994). 'Ethno-Graphics and the Moving Body', *Man*, 29, no. 4, 929–74.

Fensham, R. and Carter, A. (eds) (2011). *Dancing Naturally. Nature, Neo-Classicism and Modernity in Early Twentieth Century Dance*. Basingstoke: Palgrave Macmillan.

Fiske, J. and Hartley, J. (1993) [1978]. 'Dance as Light Entertainment'. In D. Allen and S. Jordan (eds).

Fletcher, S. (1984). *Women First. The Female Tradition in English Physical Education 1880–1980*. London: Athlone.

Flett, J. F. and Flett, T. M. (1964). *Traditional Dancing in Scotland*. London: Routledge and Kegan Paul.

—— (1979). *Traditional Step-Dancing in Lakeland*. London: English Folk Dance and Song Society.

Flitch, J. E. C. (1912). *Modern Dancing and Dancers*. London: Grant Richards.

Foster, S. L. (ed.). (1995). *Choreographing History*. Bloomington: Indiana University Press.

—— (1996). *Corporealities: Dancing, Knowledge, Culture, and Power*. London and New York: Routledge.

Foulkes, R. (1997). *Church and Stage in Victorian England*. Cambridge: Cambridge University Press.

Franks, A. H. (1963). *Social Dance: A Short History*. London: Routledge & Kegan Paul.

Gallagher, C. and Laqueur, T. (eds). (1987). *The Making of the Modern Body: Sexuality and Society in the Nineteenth Century*. Berkeley, Los Angeles and London: University of California Press.

Gammon, V. (2008). 'Many Useful Lessons: Cecil Sharp, Education and the Folk Dance Revival, 1899–1924', *Cultural and Social History*, vol. 5, 1, 75–98.

Genné, B. (1982). 'P. J. S. Richardson and the Birth of British Ballet', *Proceedings of the Fifth Annual Conference of the Society for Dance History Scholars*, 94–101.

Girouard, M. (1977). *Sweetness and Light. The 'Queen Anne' Movement 1860–1900*. Oxford: Clarendon.

—— (1981). *The Return to Camelot. Chivalry and the English Gentleman*. London and New Haven: Yale University Press.

George-Graves, N. (2009). '"Just like Being at the Zoo". Primitivity and Ragtime Dance'. In J. Malnig (2009b).

Golden, E. (2007). *Vernon and Irene Castle's Ragtime Revolution*. Lexington, Kentucky: University Press of Kentucky.

Gottschild, B. D. (2002). *Waltzing in the Dark. African American Vaudeville and Race Politics in the Swing Era*. New York and Basingstoke: Palgrave Macmillan.

Grau, A. (2005). 'When the Landscape becomes Flesh: An Investigation into Body Boundaries with Special Reference to Tiwi Dance and Western Classical Ballet', *Body and Society*, 11, no. 4, 141–63.

Green, A. (2007). *Cultural History. Theory and History*. Basingstoke: Palgrave Macmillan.

Greville, B. V. (1892). *The Gentlewoman in Society*. London: Henry & Co.

—— (1927). *Vignettes of Memory*. London: Hutchinson & Co.

Grossmith, G. [1884]. *See Me Reverse*. London: J. Bath.

—— [1887]. *See Me Dance The Polka*. London: J. Bath.

Grossmith, G. (1888). *A Society Clown. Reminiscences*. J. W. Arrowsmith's Bristol Library.

Grossmith, G. and Grossmith, W. [1892] (1999). *The Diary of a Nobody*. London: Penguin Books.

Grove, L. (1895). *Dancing*. London: Longmans, Green & Co.

Haley, B. (1978). *The Healthy Body and Victorian Culture*. Cambridge, Mass.: Harvard University Press.

Hall, C. (2000a). 'The Nation Within and Without'. In C. Hall, K. McClelland and J. Rendall.

Hall, C., McClelland, K. and Rendall, J. (2000b). *Defining the Victorian Nation. Class, Race, Gender and the Reform Act of 1867*. Cambridge: Cambridge University Press.

Hammond, S. N. (1984). 'The "Gavotte de Vestris": A Dance of Three Centuries', *Society for Dance History Scholars. Proceedings of the 7th Annual Conference*, pp. 47–52.

Harris, J. (1994). *Private Lives, Public Spirit: Britain 1870–1914*. London: Penguin.

Haskell, H. (1988). *The Early Music Revival: A History*. London: Thames and Hudson.

Heilmann, A. (1998). *The Late-Victorian Marriage Question*. 5 vols. London: Routledge.

Henderson, Mrs N. [1879]. *Etiquette of the Ball-Room and Guide to All the Fashionable Dances*. 20th edn. London: Simpkin Marshall & Co.

Hesse, C. (2004). 'The New Empiricism', *Cultural and Social History*, 1, no. 2, 201–7.

Hewitt, C. (1912). 'The Turkey Trot', *The Dancing Times*, November, 80–1.

Hindson, C. (2007). *Female Performance Practice on the Fin-de-Siècle Popular Stages of London and Paris. Experiment and Advertisement*. Manchester and New York: Manchester University Press.

Hobsbawm, E. J. (1987). *The Age of Empire: 1875–1914*. London: Weidenfeld and Nicolson.
Holt, A. [1879]. *Fancy Dresses Described. Or, What to Wear at Fancy Balls*. London: *The Queen*.
—— (1907). *How to Dance the Revived Ancient Dances*. London: Horace Cox.
Holt, R. (2006). 'The Amateur Body and the Middle-Class Man: Work, Health and Style in Victorian Britain', *Sport in History*, 26, 3, 352–69.
Honey, J. R. de. S. (1977). *Tom Brown's Universe. The Development of the Victorian Public School*. London: Millington.
Hook, P. and Poltimore, M. (1986). *Popular 19th Century Painting. A Dictionary of European Genre Painters*. Woodbridge, Suffolk: Antique Collectors' Club.
Horn, P. (1992). *High Society. The English Social Élite, 1880–1914*. Stroud, Gloucestershire: Alan Sutton.
Houfe, S. (2002). *Phil May: His Life and Work 1864–1903*. Aldershot: Ashgate.
Humphrey E. [1874]. *London Ball Room Guide*. London: Joseph Williams.
Humphrey, W. (1911a). 'Can You Do The One-Step?', *The Dancing Times*, January, 80–1.
—— (1911b). 'The Double Boston', *The Dancing Times*, October, 8–9.
—— (1911c). 'The Two-Step', *The Dancing Times*, November, 32–3.
Humphry, Mrs C. E. [1897a]. *Manners for Men*. London: Ward, Lock & Co.
—— [1897b]. *Manners for Women*. London: Ward, Lock & Co.
Hyatt-Woolf, E. (1911). 'Passing of the Waltz', *The Dance Journal*, May, 5–6.
Hyman, A. (1975). *The Gaiety Years*. London: Cassell.
International Encyclopedia of Dance (1998). Oxford: Oxford University Press.
Isaac, B. (1992). *The British Association of Teachers of Dancing. A Brief Review of One Hundred Years*. Glasgow: The British Association of Teachers of Dancing.
ISTD (Imperial Society of Teachers of Dancing) (2004). *100 Years of Dance. A History of the ISTD Examinations Board*. London: ISTD Dance Examinations Board.
Jackson, L. and Nathan, Lee. (2004). *Victorian London*. London: New Holland.
Jacotot, S. (2007). 'The Inversion of Social Dance Transfers between Europe and the Americas at the Turn of the Twentieth Century', *Choreographies of Migration. Patterns of Global Mobility 2007 Conference Proceedings Congress on Research in Dance*, 106–111.
James, L. (2006). *The Middle Class. A History*. London: Abacus.
Järvinen, H. (2008). '"The Russian Barnum": Russian Opinions on Diaghilev's Ballets Russes, 1909–1914', *Dance Research*, 26, no. 1, 18–41.
Jennings, C. (2007). *Them and Us. The American Invasion of British High Society*. Stroud, Gloucestershire: Sutton.
Johnson, A. E. (1915). *The Russian Ballet*. London: Constable & Co.
Jones, C. (2004). 'Peter Mandler's "Problem with Cultural History", or, is Playtime Over?' *Cultural and Social History*, 1, no. 2, 209–15.
Jupp, J. (1923). *The Gaiety Stage Door. Thirty Years' Reminiscences of the Theatre*. London: Jonathan Cope.
Kaplan, J. H. and Booth, M. R. (eds). (1996). *The Edwardian Theatre. Essays on Performance and the Stage*. Cambridge: Cambridge University Press.
Katz, R. (1973). 'The Egalitarian Waltz', *Comparative Studies in Society and History*, 15, 3, 368–77.

Koda, H. and Bolton, A. (2007). *Poiret*. New York: Metropolitan Museum of Art, New Haven, Conn., and London: Yale University Press.

Kealiinohomoku, J. W. (1969–70). 'An Anthropologist Looks at Ballet as a Form of Ethnic Dance', *Impulse*, 24–33.

Kehoe, E. (2004). *The Titled Americans. Three American Sisters and the British Aristocratic World into Which They Married*. New York: Atlantic Monthly Press.

Kelly, R. M. (1996). *The Art of Georges du Maurier*. Aldershot: Scolar Press.

Keppel, S. R. (1958). *Edwardian Daughter*. London: Hamish Hamilton.

Kift, D. (1996). *The Victorian Music Hall. Culture, Class and Conflict*. Cambridge: Cambridge University Press.

Kinney, T. and Kinney, M. W. (1914). *The Dance: Its Place in Art and Life*. London: William Heinemann.

Koritz, A. (1996). 'Re/Moving Boundaries: From Dance History to Cultural Studies'. In G. Morris (ed.).

Knowles, M. (2009). *The Wicked Waltz and Other Scandalous Dances. Outrage at Couple Dancing in the 19th and Early 20th Centuries*. Jefferson, North Carolina, and London: McFarlane & Co.

Kuchta, D. (1996). 'The Making of the Self-Made Man: Class, Clothing and English Masculinity, 1688–1832'. In V. De Grazia with E. Furlough.

Lamb, W. [1896]. *Everybody's Guide to Ball-Room Dancing*. London: W. R. Russell & Co.

Langford, P. (2000). *Englishness Identified. Manners and Character 1650–1850*. Oxford: Oxford University Press.

Lawson, E. (1874). *A Brief Essay on Dancing and its Refining Influence in Social Life with Practical Remarks*. London: H. K. Lewis.

LeBlanc, É. [1883]. *Companion to the Ball Room and Self-Instructor in the Art of Dancing*. London: The Author.

Ledbetter, K. (2009). *British Victorian Women's Periodicals*. Basingstoke: Palgrave Macmillan.

Lennard, J. C. (1911). 'Ball-Room Dancing of To-day', *Dancing Times*, April, 164–5.

Leppert, R. (1988). *Music and Image. Domesticity, Ideology and Socio-Cultural Formation in Eighteenth-Century England*. Cambridge: Cambridge University Press.

Lounger in Society, The (1881). *The Glass of Fashion. A Universal Handbook of Social Etiquette and Home Culture for Ladies and Gentlemen*. London: John Hogg.

Lovelace, Countess (1932). 'Society and the Season'. In Contributors, Twenty-Seven.

Lowenthal, D. (1985). *The Past is a Foreign Country*. Cambridge: Cambridge University Press.

Lowerson, J. (1993). *Sport and the English Middle Class 1870–1914*. Manchester: Manchester University Press.

——— (2005). *Amateur Operatics. A Social and Cultural History*. Manchester: Manchester University Press.

Machray, R. (1902). *The Night Side of London*. London: John Macqueen.

Macintosh, F. (ed.). (2010). *The Ancient Dancer in the Modern World. Responses to Greek and Roman Dance*. Oxford: Oxford University Press.

Macqueen-Pope, W. (1949). *Gaiety. Theatre of Enchantment*. London: W. H. Allen.

———— (1956). *Nights of Gladness*. London: Hutchinson.

McCrone, K. (1993). '"Playing the Game" and "Playing the Piano": Physical Culture and Culture at Girls' Public Schools, c. 1850–1914'. In G. Walford.

McGowan, M. (2008). *Dance in the Renaissance: European Fashion, French Obsession*. London and New Haven: Yale University Press.

McIntosh, P. (1968). *Physical Education in England since 1800*. London: G. Bell and Sons.

McKeon, M. (ed.). (2000). *Theory of the Novel. A Critical Approach*. Baltimore and London: John Hopkins University Press.

McMains, J. (2006). *Glamour Addiction. Inside the American Ballroom Dance Industry*. Middletown, Connecticut: Wesleyan University Press.

Malcolm, I. (1932). 'Gilded Youth'. In Contributors, Twenty-Seven.

Malnig, J. (1992). *Dancing Till Dawn: A Century of Exhibition Ballroom Dance*. New York and London: New York University Press.

———— (2009a). 'Apaches, Tangos, and Other Indecencies. Women, Dance, and New York Nightlife of the 1910s'. In J. Malnig.

———— (ed.) (2009b). *Ballroom, Boogie, Shimmy Sham, Shake. A Social and Popular Dance Reader*. Urbana and Chicago: University of Illinois Press.

Mandler, P. (2004a). 'The Problem with Cultural History', *Cultural and Social History* 1, no. 1, 94–117.

———— (2004b). 'Problems in Cultural History: A Reply', *Cultural and Social History*, 1, no. 3, 326–32.

———— (2006). *The English National Character. The History of an Idea from Edmund Burke to Tony Blair*. New Haven and London: Yale University Press.

Mangan, J. A. (2008). *Athleticism in the Victorian and Edwardian Public School: The Emergence and Consolidation of an Educational Ideology*. Cambridge: Cambridge University Press.

Mangan J. A. and Walvin, J. (eds). (1987). *Manliness and Morality. Middle-Class Masculinity in Britain and America, 1800–1940*. Manchester: Manchester University Press.

Mansfield, A. and Cunnington, P. (1973). *Handbook of English Costume in the Twentieth Century, 1900–1950*. London: Faber and Faber.

Marquis and Clayton, Miss. [1913]. *How to Dance the Tango*. London: George Newnes.

Marryat, F. (1841). *Olla Podrida*. Paris: A. & W. Galignani.

Melrose, C. J. [n.d.]. *Dancing Up to Date. Ball Room Dancing Taught On Scientific Principles*. London: Hart & Co. (copy in Library of the ISTD, London).

Mendes V. D. and De La Haye, A. (2009). *Lucile. London, Paris, New York and Chicago 1890s–1930s*. London: V & A Publishing.

Michel, A. (1945). 'Kate Vaughan or the Poetry of the Skirt Dance', *Dancing Times*, January, 12–13, 29–32.

Mill, J. S. (1869). *The Subjection of Women*. New York: D. Appleton & Co.

Moers, E. (1960). *The Dandy. Brummell to Beerbohm*. London: Secker and Warburg.

Morgan, M. (1994). *Manners, Morals and Class in England, 1774–1858*. Basingstoke: Macmillan.

Morris, G. (ed.). (1996). *Moving Words, Re-writing Dance*. London: Routledge.

———— (2009). 'Dance Studies/Cultural Studies', *Dance Research Journal*, 41, 1, 82–100.

Mouvet, M. [1915]. *Maurice's Art of Dancing*. New York: Schirmer.

Murphy, S. (1985). *The Duchess of Devonshire's Ball*. London: Sidgwick and Jackson.

Naylor, S. (1913). *Gaiety and George Grossmith. Random Reflections on the Serious Business of Enjoyment*. London: Stanley Paul.

Nead, L. (2000). *Victorian Babylon. People, Streets and Images in Nineteenth-Century London*. New Haven & London: Yale University Press.

Neal, M. (1910). *The Esperance Morris Book*. London: J Curwen & Sons.

Nevill, R. (1912). *The Man of Pleasure*. London: Chatto & Windus.

——— (1919). *Echoes Old and New*. London: Chatto & Windus.

Newton, S. M. (1974). *Health, Art & Reason. Dress Reformers of the Nineteenth Century*. London: John Murray.

Nickalls, G. O. (1958). 'You Should have Seen us Dance the Polka', *The Queen*, 21 January, pp. 28–9.

Nott, J. (2002). *Music for the People. Popular Music and Dance in Interwar Britain*. Oxford: Oxford University Press.

Osborne, P. (1992). 'Modernity is a Qualitative, Not a Chronological Category', *New Left Review*, 192, 65–84.

Parsonage, C. (2005). *The Evolution of Jazz in Britain, 1880–1935*. Aldershot: Ashgate.

Pascoe, C. E. (1879). *Schools for Girls and Colleges for Women. A Handbook of Female Education Chiefly Designed for the Use of Persons of the Upper Middle Class*. London: Hardwick & Bogue.

——— (1897). *The London Season. The Monthly Edition of 'London of Today'*. N.S.3, no. 25, May. London: Benrose & Sons.

Pearce, D. [1986] (2001). *London's Mansions. The Palatial Houses of the Nobility*. London: B. T. Batsford.

Peck, W. (1952). *A Little Learning. Or, A Victorian Childhood*. London: Faber & Faber.

Peel, B. (1986). *Dancing and Social Assemblies in York in the Eighteenth and Nineteenth Centuries* Guildford, Surrey: National Resource Centre for Dance, University of Surrey.

Pells, R. (1997). *Not Like Us. How Europeans Have Loved, Hated, and Transformed American Culture Since World War II*. New York: Basic Books.

Penny, P. (1999). 'Dancing at the Interface of the Social and Theatrical. Focus on the Participatory Patterns of Contemporary Competitive Ballroom Dancing', *Dance Research*, 17, no. 1, 47–74.

Perkin, H. (1989). *The Rise of Professional Society. England since 1880*. London and New York: Routledge.

Perugini, M. E. (1915). *The Art of Ballet*. London: Martin Seeker.

Pickering, M. (2008). *Blackface Minstrelsy in Britain*. Aldershot, Hampshire: Ashgate.

Powell, V. (1978). *Margaret, Countess of Jersey. A Biography*. London: Heinemann.

Platt, L. (2004). *Musical Comedy on the West End Stage, 1890–1939*. Basingstoke: Palgrave Macmillan.

Pugh, M. (1999). *State and Society: British and Political History, 1870–1997*. 2nd edn. London: Hodder Arnold.

Quirey, B. (1976). *May I Have the Pleasure? The Story of Popular Dancing*. London: BBC Books.

Quirey, B. and Holmes, M. (1970). 'Apology for History. The Great Divide: Misrepresentations', *The Dancing Times*, June, 485–86.

Ralph, R. (1985). *The Life and Works of John Weaver*. London: Dance Books.

Rappaport, E. D. (2001). 'Travelling in the Lady Guides' London: Consumption, Modernity and the *Fin de Siècle* Metropolis'. In M. J. Daunton and B. Rieger (eds).

Readman, P. (2005). 'The Place of the Past in English Culture c. 1890–1914', *Past and Present*, 186, 147–99.

Richardson, P. J. S. [1910]. *The Americans' Mecca. Paris and the Beautiful Land of France*. London: T. M. Middleton.

—— (1946). *A History of English Ballroom Dancing (1910–1945)*. London: Herbert Jenkins.

—— (1960). *The Social Dances of the Nineteenth Century in England*. London: Herbert Jenkins.

Richardson, C. S., Lady. (1913). *Dancing, Beauty and Games*. London: Arthur L. Humphreys.

Ripman, O. (1974). 'Wordy', *Dancing Times*, July, 581; 'Steps in Time', *The Dancing Times*, August, 639.

Robinson, D. (2004). *Race in Motion: Reconstructing the Practice, Profession, and Politics of Social Dancing, New York City 1900–1930*. PhD, University of California, Riverside.

—— (2006). '"Oh, You Black Bottom!": Appropriation, Authenticity and Opportunity in the Jazz Dance Teaching of 1920s New York', *Dance Research Journal*, 38, nos 1/2, 19–42.

—— (2009). 'Performing American: Ragtime Dancing as Participatory Minstrelsy', *Dance Chronicle*, 32, 1, 89–126.

—— (2010). 'The Ugly Duckling: The Refinement of Ragtime Dancing and the Mass Production and Marketing of Modern Social Dance', *Dance Research*, 28, 2, 179–99.

Rogers, E. A. (2003). *The Quadrille. A Practical Guide to its Origin, Development and Performance*. Orpington: C. & E. Rogers.

Rubin, M. (2002). 'What is Cultural History Now?' In D. Cannadine (ed.).

Russell, T. and Bourassa, D. (2007). *The Menuet de la Cour*. Hildesheim, Zürich and New York: Georg Olms Verlag.

Ruyter, N. L. C. (1979). *Reformers and Visionaries: The Americanization of the Art of Dance*. New York: Dance Horizons.

St. George, A. (1993). *The Descent of Manners. Etiquette, Rules and the Victorians*. London: Chatto & Windus.

St. Johnston, R. (1906). *A History of Dancing*. London: Simpkin, Marshall. Hamilton, Kent & Co.

Savigliano, M. E. (1995). *Tango and the Political Economy of Passion*. Oxford: Westview Press.

Scott, E. [1885]. *The Art of Waltzing and Guide to the Ball-Room*. London: Hart Co.

—— (1887a). *Dancing As It Should Be. For Learners, Dancers and All Readers*. London: Frederick Pitman.

—— (1887b). *Grace and Folly. Or Dancing and Dancers*. London: Ward and Downey.

—— (1888). *The Waltz at a Glance*. London: Francis Bros & Day.

—— (1892). *Dancing as an Art and Pastime*. London: George Bell & Sons.

—— (1899). *Dancing in All Ages*. London: Swan Sonnenschein & Co.

—— (1911). *Dancing*. London: G. Bell & Sons.

—— (1913). *All About the Boston. A Critical and Practical Treatise on Modern Waltz Variations*. London: George Routledge & Sons.

——(1920). *Dancing Artistic and Social*. London: G. Bell and Sons.

Searle, G. R. (2004). *A New England? Peace and War 1886–1918*. Oxford: Clarendon Press.

Seeley, R. and Bunnett, R. (1989). *London Musical Shows on Record 1889–1989*. Harrow: Gramophone.

Sharp, C. J. (1907–13). *The Morris Book*, 5 parts. London: Novello.

Sheafe, A. (1913). *The Fascinating Boston: How to Dance and to Teach the Popular New Social Favorite*. Boston: Boston Music Co.

Silvester, V. (1958). *Dancing is My Life: An Autobiography*. London: Heinemann.

Silvester, V. and Richardson, P. J. S. (1936). *The Art of the Ballroom*. London: Herbert Jenkins.

Sinfield, A. (1994). *The Wilde Century. Effeminacy, Oscar Wilde and the Queer Moment*. New York: Cassell.

Slobin, M. (1993). *Subcultural Sounds. Micromusics of the West*. Middletown, CT: Wesleyan University Press.

Solie, R. A. (2004). *Music in Other Words. Victorian Conversations*. Berkeley, Los Angeles and London: University of California Press.

Spencer, H. (1861). *Education: Intellectual, Moral and Physical*. London: Williams and Norgate.

—— (1950). *Literary Style and Music. Including Two Short Essays on Gracefulness and Beauty*. London: Watts & Co.

Stearns, M. and Stearns, J. (1968). *Jazz Dance. The Story of American Vernacular Dance*. New York: Schirmer Books.

Stewart, E. V. T., Marchioness of Londonderry (1938). *Retrospect*. London: Frederick Muller.

Stock, J. (1998). 'New Musicologies, Old Musicologies: Ethnomusicology and the Study of Western Music', *Current Musicology*, 62, 40–68.

Summers, L. (2003). *Bound to Please: A History of the Victorian Corset*. 2nd edn. Oxford: Berg.

Taddei, A. (1999). 'London Clubs in the Late Nineteenth Century', *Economics Discussion Papers in Economic and Social History*, 28, University of Oxford, http://www.nuff.ox.ac.uk/economics/history/paper28/28taddeiweb1.pdf. Accessed 11 June 2010.

Temperley, N. (ed.) (1989). *The Lost Chord: Essays on Victorian Music*. Bloomington, Indiana: Indiana University Press.

Thomas, A. (ed.). (1992). *A New and Most Excellent Dancing Master. The Journal of Joseph Lowe's Visits to Balmoral and Windsor (1852–1860) to Teach Dance to the Family of Queen Victoria*. Stuyvesant, New York: Pendragon Press.

Thomas, H. (2003). *The Body, Dance and Cultural Theory*. Basingstoke: Palgrave Macmillan.

Thompson, A. (1998). *Dancing through Time: Western Social Dance in Literature 1400–1918. Selections*. Jefferson, N.C; London: McFarland.

Thompson, F. M. L. (1988). *The Rise of Respectable Society. A Social History of Britain, 1830–1900*. London: Fontana.

Thorold, P. (2001). *The London Rich. The Creation of a Great City*. London: Penguin.

Thorpe, J. (1935). *English Illustration. The Nineties.* London: Faber & Faber.

Tickner, L. (2000). *Modern Life and Modern Subjects. British Art in the Early Twentieth Century.* London and New Haven: Yale University Press.

Tombs, R. and Tombs, I. (2006). *That Sweet Enemy. The French and the British from the Sun King to the Present.* London: William Heinemann.

Tomko, L. J. (1999). *Dancing Class: Gender, Ethnicity, and Social Divides in American Dance, 1890–1920.* Bloomington, Indiana: Indiana University Press.

Tosh, J. (1999). *A Man's Place. Masculinity and the Middle-Class Home in Victorian England.* New Haven and London: Yale University Press.

——— (2005a). 'Masculinities in an Industrializing Society: Britain, 1800–1914', *Journal of British Studies,* 44, 2, 330–42.

——— (2005b). *Manliness and Masculinities in Nineteenth-Century Britain. Essays on Gender, Family and Empire.* London: Pearson Education.

Trollope, A. (1875). *The Way We Live Now.* Leipzig: Bernhard Tauchnitz.

Urlin, E. L. [1914]. *Dancing Ancient and Modern.* London: Simpkin, Marshall, Hamilton, Kent & Co.

Vann, J. D. and VanArsdel, R. T. (eds) (1994). *Victorian Periodicals and Victorian Society.* Toronto: University of Toronto Press.

Vicinus, M. (ed.) (1972). *Suffer and Be Still. Women in the Victorian Age.* Bloomington & London: Indiana University Press.

——— (1977). *A Widening Sphere. Changing Roles of Victorian Women.* Bloomington & London: Indiana University Press.

——— (1985). *Independent Women. Work and Community for Single Women 1850– 1920.* London: Virago.

Vuillier, G. (1898). *A History of Dancing. From the Earliest Ages to Our Own Times.* London: William Heinemann.

Wagner, A. (1997). *Adversaries of Dance. From the Puritans to the Present.* Urbana: University of Illinois Press.

Walford, G. (ed.). (1993). *The Private Schooling of Girls. Past and Present.* London: Woburn Press.

Walker, C. B. (2001). '"The Triumph" in England, Scotland and the United States', *Folk Music Journal,* 8, 1, 4–40.

Walker, K. S. (2007). 'The Espinosas: A Dancing Dynasty', *Dance Chronicle,* 30, 2, 447–76.

Walton, J. K. (1983). *The English Seaside Resort: A Social History 1750–1914.* Leicester: Leicester University Press.

Walton, J. K. and Walvin, J. (eds) (1983). *Leisure in Britain 1780–1939.* Manchester: Manchester University Press.

Walvin, J. (1973). *Black and White. The Negro and English Society, 1555–1945.* London: Allen Lane.

Washabaugh, W. (ed.) (1998). *The Passion of Music and Dance: Body, Gender, and Sexuality.* New York and Oxford: Berg.

Watts, C. (2004). 'Thinking about the X Factor, or, What's the Cultural History of Cultural History?', *Cultural and Social History,* 1, no. 2, 217–24.

Weaver, J. (1712). *An Essay towards An History of Dancing, etc.* London.

White, J. (2007). *London in the Nineteenth Century.* London: Jonathan Cape.

Wiener, M. J. (1981). *English Culture and the Decline of the Industrial Spirit, 1850–1920.* Cambridge: Cambridge University Press.

Williams, S. M. (1892). *Round London. Down East and Up West.* London: Macmillan.

Wilson, C. A. (2009). *Literature and Dance in Nineteenth-Century Britain. Jane Austin to the New Woman*. Cambridge: Cambridge University Press.

Wilson, E. (2003). *Adorned in Dreams. Fashion and Modernity*. London: I. B. Tauris.

Woodcock, S. C. (1989). 'Margaret Rolfe's Memoirs of Marie Taglioni: Part 1', *Dance Research*, 7, no. 1, 3–19. Part 2, *Dance Research*, 7, no. 2, 55–69.

Woolf, V. (1924) (2000). 'Mr. Bennett and Mrs Brown'. In M. McKeon.

X, Countess of. (1932). *Society through the Hoop*. London: T. Werner Laurie.

Young, L. (2003). *Middle-Class Culture in the Nineteenth Century. America, Australia and Britain*. Basingstoke: Palgrave Macmillan.

Index

Notes on the index: References to illustrations are in bold. Typically, an individual name falls under the subject heading. For example, the Turkey Trot is under Dances (types of) and the Savoy is under Hotels.

Adelaide, Mme, 87, 91
Advertisements, 17, 18, 41, 75, 78, 83–4, 86, 87, 88, 148, 156, 158, 183, 186
Alexandre, Monsieur, 83
Almanos, Los, 155, 163, 180
American Dancing Masters Association, 167
American War of Independence, 23, 138
Americans, 33, 34, 37, 65, 98, 101, 107, 146, 150, 167, 168–9, 177–8
see also dances (types of)
Anastasia, Grand Duchess of Russia, 163
Ancaster, Countess of, 17, 26, 60, 109, 201
Anglo-Boer War, 141
Aristocracy, see Society
Armytage, Hon. Mrs, 18, 202
Armytage, Percy, 32, 202
Articled pupil system (teacher training), 86–7, 92–3
Artifice, see nature
Artists and artworks, 20, 26–7, 44, 45, 70, 71, 115, 116, 181
Asquith, Cynthia, 201
Asquith, Margot, 201
At homes, 41, 77, 111

Ballroom dancing, see dances (types of); dancing, English style of ballroom
Ballroom hold, see dancing, technique
Balls
  amenities at, 26
  boredom with repertoire of, 5, 59, 64

Caledonian, 55, 157
charity, 23, 35, 36, 39–40, 44
committees, 35–6, 42
complaints about young men at, 123, 125, 126
county, 23, 35–6, 54
court, 24–5, 27, 46, 54, 59, 72, 77, 81, 108
Covent Garden Costume, 43–4
decorations at, 22, 26, 32
Duchess of Devonshire's, 20, 44
etiquette at, 28–30, 77, 108, 118, 120, 123, 125
fancy dress, 27, 44
guests at, 22, 27, 28–9, 31, 35, 124
historical costume, 20, 27, 30, 44, 71
Hunt, 36
Inhabitants', 35
invitations and guest lists, 10, 25, 28, 31–2, 40, 174
as marriage market, 8, 28, 30, 33, 38, 95, 107, 135
masked, 30, 43
Mayor's, 35
military, 134
physical conditions at, 124
programmes (dance cards), 30–1
public, 11, 22, 36
Royal Caledonian, 36–7
royalty at, 28–9
Scottish, 49, 55
semi-public, 30, 35, 44
Society, 5, 6, 7–8, 10–11, 16, 17, 22, 24, 26, 28–32, 33, 34, 37, 47, 54, 69, 141, 160
state, 10, 24–5, 30, 47, 48, 62, 65, 72, 98, 135, 142
stewards at, 35, 36

supper at, 22, 26, 27, 30, 36, 41, 63, 123, 126, 128
young men's complaints about, 124–27
see also dances (social events); dances (types of); dancing; houses; manuals; music; rowdyism
Ballet, 48, 80, 83, 90, 93, 97, 112, 114–15, 120, 122, 145, 159
Ballets Russes, 159, 190
Bands, see music
Baynes, Sydney, 148
Berlin, Irving, 154, 167
Bishop, Sidney, 184
Bland family, 83
Bohemia, 44, 45, 150, 178, 181
Boston (dance), 67, 143, **145–8**, 155, 156, 157, 160, 161, 165, 171, 188, 189, 199
Bourgeoisie, see middle class
Bows, 47, 71, 79, 97
Bradley, Josephine, 168, 204
Brighton, 81, 82, 83, 88, 157
British Association of Teachers of Dancing (BATD), 90, 182, 184, 188
British Empire, 6, 24, 69, 75, 98, 104, 129, 133, 135, 136, 138, 176, 193, 194
Buss, Frances, 106

Cake Walk, 56, 69, 151–2, 153, 161, 184
Callisthenics, 76, 78, 83, 84, 104, 105–6
see also physical training
Castle, Vernon and Irene, 154, 155, 167, 185, 192, 205
Cellarius, 48
Cerrito, Fanny, 117
Chalif, Louis, 188
Chaperones, 22, 28, 30, 45, 109, 142, 144, 172, 180
Chaplin, Nellie, 71, 72
Charitable events, 92, 111
see also balls, charity; dances, charity
Churchill, Lady Randolph, 33, 71, 201

Civilization (concept), 95, 102, 116, 136, 169, 176, 177, 178, 180, 186, 189, 193, 195
ballroom as microcosm of, 7, 20, 29, 160, 189
fears of decline of, 69, 143, 154, 162, 173, 174, 175, 178, 195
and the past, 71, 72, 115, 116, 119, 197
see also degeneration; race and racism; rowdyism
Class, see lower class; middle class; Society
Classes, dancing, 58, 59, 66, 67, 69, 76, 77, 80, 84, 88, **91–2**, 93, 126, 130–1, 135, 148, 155, 159, 162, 166, 183
see also schools; teachers
Clothing, 7, 8, 38, 41, 42
men's, 27, 119, 124–5, 129, 133, 170, 171
women's, 17, 22, 27, 28, 33, 36, 56, 82, 92, 98, 99, 101, 102, 103, 104, 107, 112, 115, 116, 117, 163, 173–4
see also corsets; dress reform
Clubs, dancing
Keen Dancers Club (K.D.S., later Boston Club), 146, 154, 188
Public Schools and Universities Dance Club, 144, 188
Ralli-Boston Club, 157
Royalist Club, 144, 165, 184, 188
Thé Dansant Tango and Boston Club, 157
Coffin, Hayden, 134
Collier, Beatrice, 153
Competitions, dance, 184, 186, 192, 194, 195
Cornwallis West, George, 128
Corsets, 99, 101–2, 103, 104, 112, 125, 142, 173
Court presentation, 12, 79, 98–9, **100**, 141, 157, 159
Courts
British, 7, 32, 55, 72, 76, 101, 108, 165, 180, 193
French, 75, 80, 117, 120
German, 72

Courville, Albert de, 154
Cowper Coles, Alice, 72
Coyne, Joseph, 167
Crawford Flitch, J.E., 19, 153
Crompton, Robert, 18, 39, 46, 47, 49,
    52, 54, 56, 71, 72, 85, 88, 120,
    135, 156, 157, 198, 202
Crozier, Gladys Beattie, 163, 171, 173
Curtseys, 47, 71, 93, 97, 98–9, 108

Dacunha, Henri, 84, 90
D'Albert, Charles, 72, 85, 202–3
Dances (social events)
    afternoon, 27–8, 153
    assemblies, 41–2, 57, 59, 84, 141,
        155, 184, 188
    barrack or garrison, 28
    carpet, 28, 40
    charity, 38, 159, 167
    Cinderella, 38–9
    dinner, 165
    drawing room, 27–8, 85, 122, 124,
        157
    military, 28
    picnic, 42
    private, 27, 28, 37–8, 43, 171, 184
    public, 9, 38–9, 41, 43, 144
    Society, 27, 33, 171
    shilling hops, 58, 69, 151
    small and earlies, 27
    subscription, 36, 38–9, 42–3, 44,
        58, 66, 84, 144, 146, 165, 184,
        186
    supper, 165, 166
    village, 67, 69
    see also balls; clubs, dancing; dances
        (types of); dancing; manuals;
        music; venues
Dances (types of)
    adagio, 153
    African-American, 7, 11, 156, 160,
        162, 174, 176
    American, 3, 11–12, 55–6, 85, 89,
        160, 174, 175, 178, 187
    ancient Greek, 115–16
    Apache, 152–3, 154
    Barn, 55, 60, 69, 93
    Branle, 71
    Bunny Hug, 162, 175, 178, 185

Chorolistha, 85
Cotillion, 49, 122
country, 36, 54, 72, 76, 198, 199
court, 75
Furlana, 165
Galop, 36, 54, 56, 62, 93
Gavotte, 56, 71, 72, 77, 116, 117
Grizzly Bear, 162, 185
historical, 56, 70–2, 117, 198, 199
Hussars, 85
Iolanthe, 85
Irish Jig, 77, 137
Judy Walk, 162
Kensington Crawl, 67, 199
Latin-American, 143, 161, 174,
    175, 176
Liverpool Lurch, 67, 68
Maxixe, 152, 156, 165, 180
Mazurka, 56, 83
Menuet de la Cour, 72, 117, 180
Mignon, 56
Military Two-Step, 57, 142
Minuet, 10, 46, 56, 71, 72, 77,
    116, 151
Minuet Valse, 56
Pas de Quatre, 55
Pavane, 56, 71, 72, 77, 116
Ratcliffe Highway Kick, 67, 68
Sailor's Hornpipe, 77, 137
Saunter, 168
Schottische, 50, 55
Scottish, 37, 76, 93, 157
sequence, 55, 57, 142, 182, 184,
    188, 190–1, 193
Sir Roger de Coverley, 36, 54
step, 77, 114
Tao Tao, 165
Tempête, La, 54
Triumph, The, 36, 54–5
Turkey Trot, 154, 160, 162, 185
Veleta, 57, 142
Versa, 56
see also Boston; Cake Walk;
    dancing; fancy dances; Foxtrot;
    Lancers; manuals; music; One-
    Step; Polka; Quadrille; ragtime
    dances; standardization of dances;
    skirt dancing; Tango; Two-Step;
    Waltz; Washington Post

Dancing
  bodily contact while, 64–5, 120,
    143, 161, 171, 172, 181
  community, 43
  English style of ballroom, 3, 4, 12,
    148, 184, 186, 192–4, 196
  go-as-you-please, 59, 167, 169, 190
  and health, 50, 77, 92, 101, 104–5,
    112, 115, 125
  improvising while, 143, 144, 151,
    171, 173, 175, 187, 190
  injuries while, 61–2, 88
  partner, 29–30, 65, 107–8, 123,
    125–6, 171–2, 180
  poor standards of, 46, 58–62, 67,
    69, 89, 108, 123, 125–6, 175
  self-expression while, 170, 175, 180,
    186, 187, 200
  technique, 51, **52**, 54, 55, 59, 67,
    120, 146, 185, 192
  by social class, 9–10
  see also balls; clubs, dancing; dances
    (social events); dances (types of);
    manuals; men; music; rowdyism;
    standardization of dances;
    theatre; women
Dancing (journal), 18, 86, 88, 89
'Dancing man', the, 128–9
Dancing Times, The, 18, 20, 42, 59, 82,
    85, 88, 89, 144, 148, 149, 155,
    163, 167, 168, 175, 182, 183, 186,
    191, 192, 193, 195
Dare, Phyllis, 165
D'Auban, John, 71, 111
Dearly, Max, 152, 163
Debutantes, 12, 30, 98–9, 106–7, 109,
    111, 114, 199
  see also court presentation
Degeneration, 69–70, 116, 125, 175,
    180, 196, 197
  see also civilization; race and
    racism
D'Egville, James, 80
D'Egville, Louis, 79, 80, 81–2, 201,
    203
D'Egville, Louis (the younger), 45,
    72, 79, 80, **81**–2, 85, 91, **100**,
    116, 155, 180, 183, 195–6,
    201, 203

Deportment, 8, 10, 69, 170, 195
  English vs French, 79, 98, 116,
    120, 121
  female, 95, 98, 99, 103, 104, 105,
    106, 112, 116, 138, 142, 159
  male, 79, 118, 119, 120, 121
  teaching of, 75, 76, 77, 78–9, 80,
    81, 83, 84
Deslys, Gaby, 152
Dolmetsch, Mabel and Arnold, 71
D'Oyly Carte, Richard, 37
Dress reform, 101, 102–3
Drill, 78, 93, 131, 134, 188
  see also physical training
Drugget, 28, 40
Duff Gordon, Lady ('Lucile'), 173
Duncan, Isadora, 115
Duncan, Sara Jeanette, 33–4, 65

Edward, Prince of Wales, *see* King
    Edward VII
Edwardes, George, 113, 152
Eighteenth century, 18, 19, 20, 37, 55,
    70–1, 77, 87, 89, 95, 97, 102, 104,
    116–117, 118, 131, 135, 136, 137
Englishness, 12, 29, 79, 98, 116, 118,
    121, 134, 135–6, 137, 174, 176,
    177, 186, 190, 191, 193, 194
  see also dancing, English style of
    ballroom
Elssler, Fanny, 117
Erne, Countess of, 102
Esher, Viscount, 128, 202
Espinosa, Léon, 83
Etiquette, 7, 17, 33, 49, 95, 96, 97,
    119, 142
  see also balls; court presentation;
    men; manuals; women
Exhibition ballroom dancers, 20, 150,
    152, 153–4, 156–6, 161, 162, 166,
    184, 185
  see also individual people

Fancy dances, 76, 77, 78, 83, 91, 93,
    105, 110, 111–14, 137, 157
  see also skirt dancing
Fane, Lady Augusta, 114
Farren, Fred, 153
Femininity, *see* women

Fictional characters
    Grundy, Mrs, 102
    Harleth, Gwendolen *(Daniel Deronda)*, 30
    Melmotte, Augustus *(The Way We Live Now)*, 32
    Pooter, Mr *(The Diary of a Nobody)*, 40, 66
    Powderby, Lady *(An American Girl in London)*, 34
    Turveydrop *(Bleak House)*, 79, 151
First World War, 5, 7, 166–9, 187
Floors, dance, 27–8, 40, 41
Fontana, Georges, 158
Foxtrot, 165, 167–8, 169, 184, 188, 189, 190, 192
France, 3, 7, 12, 49, 69, 71, 138, 145, 158, 160, 186
    see also courts; deportment; Paris; resorts
Franks, A.H., 20–1
French Revolution, 23, 121, 138

Gaiety Girls, 114, 150, 173
Gaiety Theatre, 55, 78, 111, 112, 113, 150, 152, 165, 167
Games, *see* sports
Garratt, Elizabeth, 91, 92, 117, 203
Geary, Leonora, 18, 78, 84, 91
Gentility, 8, 9, 23, 41, 94, 96, 118, 119, 120, 133, 141, 176, 187, 193, 195, 198
Gentleman, *see* men
Gentlewoman, *see* women
Gilmer, Ernest, 87
Ginner, Ruby, 115
Grace, *see* deportment
Grahn, Lucile, 117
Greville, Lady Violet, 18, 22, 95–6, 106, 202
Grey, Sylvia, 113
Grossmith, George, 32, 40, 62, 63, 65–7, 205
Grossmith, George, Junior, 141, 165, 180–1, 205
Grove, Lilly, 13, 19, 71, 206
Guides, *see* manuals
Gymnastics, 78, 89, 93, 105–6, 108, 131, 134, 183

Harding, Isabella, 20, 156–9, 163, 167, 184, 196, 203
Harris, Augustus, 43
Healey sisters, 83
Henderson, Frances, 18, 48, 84, 90, 119, 121, 203
Henderson, Nicholas, 18, 90, 203
Hickey, F.R., 108
History, dance, 14–21, 71, 85, 196, 200
Hollingshead, John, 113
Hostesses, Society, 11, 23, 26, 29, 31, 32, 36, 37, 67, 71, 101, 107, 123, 124, 128, 133, 174, 197
Hotels, 9, 11, 37, 144, 146, 150, 153, 155, 156, 157, 160, 179
    Cecil, 37, 150
    Ritz, 11, 37, 159
    Royal Palace Hotel, 146, 155, 157
    Savoy, 11, 37, 44, 144, 150
    Waldorf, 37, 159, 188
    see also restaurants; venues, dancing
Houses, Society, 11, 22, 24–6, 27–8, 33, 38, 62
    Buckingham Palace, 24, **25**, 81
    Marlborough House, 24, 25, 54
    Montagu House, 26, 81
    Stafford House, 25, 26, 83
Hughes, Leonora, 190, **191**, 205
Hughes, Talbot, 71
Humphrey, Edward, 18, 41, 84, 88, 135, 203
Humphrey, Walter E., 85, 148, 155, 156, 203
Humphry, Mrs, 99, 123

Imperial Society of Dance Teachers (ISDT), 72, 148, 175, 178, 182, 183, 192, 193, 194, 198
Industrial Revolution, 23, 121, 138

James, Miss, 83
Jay sisters, 83
Jazz, *see* music
Johnson, Henry R., 18, 42, 203
Journals, *see* press
Joyce, Archibald, 148

Kellogg, Shirley, 154
Keppel, Alice, 101

King Edward VII, 7, 24, 25, 27, 32, 37, 38, 51, 62–3, 72, 101, 134, 142, 150, 201
King George V, 108, 143, 201

Lady, *see* women
Lamb, William, 203
Lancers, 48–9, 54, 60–2, 69, 102, 108, 109, 198
Langtry, Lilly, 101
Lawson, Edward, 84, 108
LeBlanc, Edouard, 49, 85, 90
Lennard, Janet, 146, 148, 154–5, 204
Leno, Dan, 114
Lessons, dancing, *see* classes
Levey, Ethel, 154, 167
Licensing laws, 89–90
Lind, Letty, 112, 113
London, 4, 24, 25, 37, 194
  Bayswater, 38, 66
  Blackheath, 38, 146
  Chelsea, 38
  Croydon, 146
  Ealing, 83, 146
  East End, 67
  Kensington, 38, 66, 82, 83
  Hampstead, 38, 83, 146
  Mayfair, 24, 25, 45, 80
  Notting Hill, 66
  Richmond, 38
  St James, 24, 131
  West End, 24, 33, 76
London Season, 6, 7, 8, 9, 16, 22, 23, 24, 27, 30–1, 32, 33, 35, 36, 58, 62, 72, 76–7, 98–9, 124, 174
Lower class, 4, 38, 59, 60, 67, 78, 96, 121, 122, 134, 160, 184, 186, 188, 189, 193, 198

Machray, Robert, 44, 69, 151
MacLennan, D.G., 167
Manners, Lady Diana, 107, 142
Marlborough, Duchess of, 33, 202
Marlborough Set, 24, 37
Manuals, 8, 18–19, 27, 28, 29, 38, 46, 84, 85, 119, 120, 121, 124
Marquis, Senor, 180
Masculinity, *see* men

Master/mistress of ceremonies, 42, 81, 84
May, Phil, 19, 70
McNaughton, J.D., 188
McQuoid, Percy, 71
Melrose, C.J., 62
Men
  about town, 44–5, 150, 170–1, 178–9
  attributes of a gentleman, 23, 30, 79, 118–22, 134, 135–6, 180, 194
  and chivalry, 109, 119, 135–6, 180
  and dancing, 64–5, 118–22, 123–24, 126, 128–9, 131, 133, 134–5, 137–8, 141, 171–2, 187
  dandy, 133, 170
  effeminacy, 137, 180
  London clubs of, 37, 44, 129, 131–3
  Masher, 66, 170, 171
  Knut (nut), 170, 171, **172**
  masculinity, 97, 118, 124, 129, 130, 131, 135, 136, 137–8, 171–2, 180, 188, 199
  see also clothing; dancing; deportment; physical training
Messel, Maud and Leonard, 71
Michau, Caroline D'Egville, 87, 91, 95, 104, 105, 119, 204
Michau, Isabel, 91
Michau, James Paul, 88
Michau, Sophia ('Mme Michau'), 80–1
Middle class, 3, 4, 8, 9, 10, 18, 19, 23, 27–8, 36, 38–41, 56, 67, 75, 87, 88, 89, 90, 92, 93–4, 96, 101, 104, 106, 114, 115, 118, 119, 121, 131, 133, 135, 136, 137, 138, 142, 144, 150, 152, 153, 158, 159, 171, 183
  lower-, 41, 55, 56–7, 69, 76, 90, 141–2, 151, 176, 182, 187–8, 189, 191, 193
  upper-, 3, 4, 8, 9, 12, 17, 31–2, 33, 35, 37–8, 42, 43, 65–6, 67, 69, 71, 76, 83, 84, 98, 103, 109, 111, 129, 130, 142, 143–4, 147, 155, 157, 165, 176, 184, 187, 188, 191, 193
Mistinguett, 152, 163, 184
Modernity, 4, 5, 79, 142, 143, 149, 153, 161, 181, 185, 190, 191, 193, 195–7
Monarchy, *see* royalty

Montagu, Oliver, 128
Mordkin, Mikhail, 159
Morris, Margaret, 115
Mouvet, Maurice, 153–4, 155, 165,
    184, 190, **191**, 192, 205
Mouvet, Oscar, 154, 155, 192, 205
Murat, Princess Eugène, 184
Music, 3, 11–12, 44, 59, 78, 143, 161,
    175, 178, 181, 186, 189, 190, 200
  bands, 19, 27, 28, 36, 41, 42, 45,
    59, 146, 162, 167, 168, 179, 186,
    187, 189
  jazz, 62, 168, 187, 189, 196
  musicians, 27, 84
  orchestras, 27, 82, 189
  ragtime, 7, 11, 56, 62, 143, 145,
    154, 161, 162, 167, 173, 177,
    178–80
  sheet, 19, 151, 154
  see also dances (types of)
Music hall, *see* theatre
Musical comedies, *see* theatre

Nature and naturalness, 3, 79, 97,
    102, 115, 120–21, 181, 195, 200
Nevill, Ralph, 133, 170–1
Newspapers, *see* press
New York, 3, 153, 154, 176, 186, 187,
    188, 193
Nouveaux riches, see middle class,
    upper-

One-Step, 143, 145, 155, 156, 161–2,
    167, 169, 189, 190, 192, 199

Paris, 3, 4, 7, 43, 75, 149–50, 152,
    153, 154, 155, 158, 163, 165, 166,
    173, 182, 184, 186, 187, 188
  see also France
Pas marché, 48, 49, 59
Peck, Winifred, 112
Petit, Emile, 83
Petit, Stephane, 83
Photographs, 20
Physical training, 76, 77–78, 93,
    104–6, 134
  see also callisthenics; drill;
    gymnastics; sports
Piaggio, Francis, 42, 90, 204

Picton Ellett, Mrs, 146
Poiret, Paul, 173
Polka, 11, 36, 50, 54, 56, 60, 63–4,
    93, 149
Press, 16–20, 24, 32, 40, 70, 89, 102,
    107, 111, 124, 129, 146, 151,
    161, 162, 165, 169, 174, 180,
    187, 190, 192
  see also Dancing Times, The;
    Dancing (journal); Punch;
    Times, The
Primrose League, 39, 67, 69
Prince of Wales, *see* King Edward VII
Punch, 19, 63, 67, **68**, 125, 126, 129,
    132, 134, **145**, 162, 171, **172**,
    173–4, 175, **179**, 187

Quadrille, 3, 9, 10, 11, 29, 32, 37, 45,
    46–9, 54, 56, 58–9, 60–1, 70, 77,
    108, 126, 142, 143
  Caledonians, 49
  First Set of, 46–7
  Floral, **61**
  Highland, 36–7
  Nationale, La, 49, 85
  Polo, 49
  Poudré, 37
  Prince Imperial's, 49
  waltzing at corners during, 59
  see also Lancers
Queen Alexandra, 25, 27, 38, 54, 62,
    63, 128, 142, 201
Queen Anne Movement, 71–2
Queen Mary, 99, 142, 143, 165, 201
Queen Victoria, 25, 44, 62, 80, 82–3,
    98, 99, 141
Quiller Orchardson, Sir William, 70

Race and racism, 5, 102, 138, 151–2,
    160, 162, 175–7, 180–1, 185–6,
    189, 196, 198, 199
Ragtime dances, 3, 17, 143, 154, 160,
    161, 162, 173, 174, 180, 181,
    185, 199
  see also music, ragtime; race and
    racism
Raven-Hill, Leonard, 178, **179**
Ray, Gabrielle, 152
Renaissance Dance Troupe, 71

Repertoire, *see* balls; dances (social events); dances (types of)
Reske, Jean de, 165
Resorts, holiday, 9, 145–6, 150, 157, 163, 184
Restaurants, 37, 38, 69, 143, 150, 152, 153, 155, 156, 161, 163
see also hotels; venues, dancing
Rhynal, Camille De, 152, 163, 184, 205
Richardson, Philip J.S., 20, 21, 49, 56, 57, 148, 154, 156, 157, 161, 166, 167, 169, 182, 183, 184, 185, 186, 187, 188, 189, 190–2, 193, 195, 206
Ripman, Olive, 92, 93, 105
Rolfe, Margaret, 80, 97, 98, 99, 105, 117, 202
Rowdyism, 49, 58–63, 67, 108, 125, 187
Royalty, 6, 9, 24, 62–3, 75, 76, 77, 80, 82, 114, 138
see also courts
Russell, Countess of, 114

Scholarship, dance, 13–16, 197
Schools, dancing, 86–8, 89
London Academy of Dancing, 84, 88, 155
South Kensington School of Dancing, 87
see also classes; teachers
Schools, private girls', 103, 106, 112
Schools, public boys', 129–31, 135, 136
Scott, Edward, 19, 29, 46, 48, 50–1, 52, 54, 56, 60, 64, 67, 69, 71–2, 75, 85, 87, 88, 91, 102, 103, 104–5, 108–9, 110, 113, 116, 121, 122, 125, 126, 128, 137, 148, 175, 179–80, 189, 192, 196, 198, 204
'See Me Dance the Polka', 63
'See Me Reverse', 65–66
Sharp, Cecil, 19, 72
Silvester, Victor, 158–9, 205
Sinden, Topsy, 113
Skirt dancing, 20, 77, 93, 108, 111–113

Social mobility, 8, 10, 23, 31–2, 33, 149, 162
Social pretensions, 40, 69
Society, 3, 4, 6–8, 9, 10, 11, 16, 17, 18, 22–4, 31–3, 34, 35, 36, 37, 43, 44–5, 46, 56, 59, 64–5, 66, 67, 69–70, 78, 90, 95, 96, 98, 101, 108, 109, 111, 114, 115, 116, 124, 129, 130, 131, 133, 142, 144, 150, 151, 152, 153, 156, 171, 173, 174, 176, 178, 184, 188, 193, 197, 198, 199
see also balls, Society; dances, Society; hostesses, Society; middle class, upper-
Sousa, John Philip, 55, 56, 151
Soutten, Mme, 90
Spencer, Herbert, 104, 115
Sports and other physical activities, 89, 93, 102, 103, 106, 109, 124, 125, 130, 131, 134, 135, 136, 188
see also callisthenics; drill; gymnastics; physical training
Stage, the, *see* theatre
Stainton Taylor, Elizabeth, 87, 91, 92, 203, 204
Standardization of dances, 182, 185, 186–93
Stewart-Richardson, Lady Constance, 114, 202
St Johnston, Reginald, 19, 61
St Maine, M. 83
Stone, Marcus, 71
Stratton, Eugene, 151
Stuart, Leslie, 151
Suzette, 154, 155, 205

Taglioni, Marie, 79–80, 90, 91, 97–9, 105, 115, 117, 201, 202, 203, 204
Tango, 3, 11, 20, 143, 152, 153, 155, 156, **158**, 160, 163–6, 171–2, 173, 180, 184, 188, 189, 192, 199
Tango teas, 155, 163, **164**, 166, 171
Taylor, Cecil, 178
Teachers, dancing, 8, 17, 33, 41, 46, 48, 75–85, 86–94, 104–5, 111, 116–17, 120, 122, 126, 146, 154–9, 161, 165, 193, 194, 195–6, 197, 198
1920–1 conferences of, 189, 190–2

Teachers, dancing – *continued*
  accreditation of, 183
  assistant, 86–7, 91, 92–3, 157,
    158–9
  competition among, 88
  as composers of dances, 47, 49,
    56–7, 84, 85, 90, 182, 188
  curriculum of, 76–8, 84, 93
  hierarchy among, 76
  as musicians, 19, 82, 87
  Paris visits of, 75–6
  poorly qualified, 88, 89, 156
  professional dancers as, 76, 80, 83,
    155–6
  publications of, 18–19, 85
  Society, 75–77, 79–83, 90, 91–2,
    156, 189
  threats to livelihood of, 88–9, 166
  training of, 86–7, 92–3, 183
  see also classes; schools; teaching;
    individual people
Teachers' Registration Council, 183
Teaching, dance, 167
  associations, 57, 89, 90, 142, 166,
    182–4, 195
  feminization of, 90–4, 183
  professionalization of, 89–90, 183
  see also British Association of
    Teachers of Dancing; classes;
    Imperial Society of Dance
    Teachers; schools; teachers
Theatre, 13–14, 19, 28, 83, 88, 92, 94,
    114, 149, 150–1, 152, 153, 154,
    155, 156, 160, 162, 165, 167, 173,
    177, 178, 185
  5064 Gerrard, 167
  Carmen Up to Data, 112
  celebrities, 20, 142, 151, 161, 184,
    194
  A Day in Paris, 153
  Hullo Ragtime, 154
  In Dahomey, 151
  Lady Madcap, 152
  The Merry Widow, 152, 154
  The Sunshine Girl, 165
  To-night's the Night, 167
  Watch Your Step, 167
  see also ballet; dances (types of);
    exhibition ballroom dancers;

Gaiety Girls; Gaiety Theatre;
    teachers
Thés dansants, 155, 157, 163, 173
Thomas, Janet, 155
Times, The, 3, 16–17, 27, 83, 86, 160,
    174, 176, 203, 204
Tissot, James, 20
Two-Step, 45, 56, 89, 141, 145, 155,
    161, 173, 199

Upper class, *see* Society
Upper Ten, *see* Society
Upton, Thomas, 90
Urlin, Ethel, 19

Vacani, Marguerite, 155, 204
Valois, Ninette de, 82
Vandyck, Alice, 155, 166
Vaughan, Kate, 55, 111–12, 113, 205
Venues, dancing, 11, 35, 37, 38–9, 40,
    41–2, 44, 143–4, 150, 165, 188
  400 Club (Embassy Club), 165, 167
  Carlton, 69, 144
  Cavendish Rooms, 19, 41, 84
  Connaught Rooms, 144
  Empress Rooms (Royal Palace
    Hotel), 42, 146, 155, 157, 158,
    159
  Grafton Galleries, 144, 146, 179,
    181, 189, 190
  Holborn Town Hall, 19, 42, 61, 69
  Kensington Town Hall, 39, 92
  Mansion House, 40
  Murray's Club, 165, **168**, 169
  palais de danse, 189, 193
  Portman Rooms, 19, 38, 39–40, 42
  Queens Gate Hall, 92, 111
  supper clubs, 165, 166
  Willis's Rooms, 36, 38
  see also hotels; houses; restaurants
Vincent, Cornelia, 91, 93

Wallflowers, 28, 107, 136, 170
Walton, Florence, 155, 165, 205
Waltz, 3, 9, 10, 11, 45, 49–**53**, 54, 56,
    58, 59, 60, 62, 63, 67, **68**, 72, 84,
    93, 101, 120, 141, 142, 143, 152,
    153, 156, 161, 169, 172, 180, 184,
    187, 189, 192, 198

Apache, 152, 153
Cotillion, 49
Hesitation, 167, 189
Hop, 67
Ju Jitsu, 152
reversing during, 64–6
Spring, 67
Valse à deux temps, 50, 51, 54, 62
Valse à trois temps, 50–1, 54, **81**
see also Boston (dance)
Washington Post, 55–6, 60, 69, 89, 93
Women
attributes of a lady, 23, 78, 79,
    95–9, 108, 109, 112, 114, 116
blue-stocking, 96, 104–5
and dancing, 69, 93, 95, 97, 107–9,
    111–17, 127, 131, 138

femininity, 96, 97, 106, 113, 142,
    150, 173
ideal body shape of, 99, 101, 102,
    103, 142, 173, 174
New, 96, 103, 109
performances by Society, 111, 114,
    117
see also clothing; dancing;
    debutantes; deportment; physical
    training
Wilson, Thomas, 50
Woolf, Virginia, 11
Wordsworth, Mrs, 78, 79, 82–3, 91,
    92–3, 105, 114, 115–16, 155, 159,
    195–6, 201, 204
Working class, *see* lower class
Wright, Fanny, 83